# About Dave Draper

"What separates Dave Draper from others of his ilk is the clarity of his prose and the directness and simplicity of his approach. Dave Draper is not a bodybuilding star who stands apart. He is the "everyman of bodybuilding" and he wants every man (and woman) to transform his (or her) life through resistance weight training. It is impossible to read Draper and not start packing your gym bag. He's the Pied Piper of bodybuilding!"

—*Ronald L. Dobrin, founding editor, East West Journal*

"Dave Draper has been a constant source of instruction, inspiration and motivation for me and countless others from all walks of life. Whatever your profession, whatever your present fitness level, the Blond Bomber can help you get the body you've always wanted, but never thought you could."

—*Paul Wagner, Lutheran pastor*

"Dave Draper sets the standard in bodybuilding as a way of life, not just a diversion from it. He speaks profoundly through his writings, though it's his action that is the real communicator. His books are simply an expression of his living example."

—*Vince McConnell, sports conditioning specialist*

"In these times of false fitness prophets and gobbledygook gurus, none of whom appear healthy—much less fit—it's refreshing to have a true fitness professional of Dave Draper's stature step forward to lead by example and expertise."

—*Jim Ganley, fitness consultant, Bow, N.H.*

"In a world of copycats, Dave is a 100% original creation. When it was far from hip to be a bodybuilder, he quite simply became one of the best the world had ever seen. Later, when it became not only hip but potentially highly profitable to be a top bodybuilder, he walked away from the hype and "scene" of it all, returning to the serenity and purity of the movement and work for its own sake and its own inherent rewards. Dave now offers the lessons and teachings of a lifetime in the gym with the wisdom and patience of a true master of the discipline. With the volumes of words written on the subject, none so clearly impart his insights from the soul or with such delight in the work, play, love and philosophy of the world of iron."

—*William H. Luttrell, Esq., B.A., J.D.*

## About Draper's *Brother Iron, Sister Steel*

"This book is an inspiration... one of the best iron sport-related books I have ever read."

—*Dr. Ken Leistner, international strength coach*

"Marvelous new book... for average folks who want to put weight lifting in their lives."

—*Eric Schoeck, KUSP, National Public Radio*

"Absolutely refreshing! With a unique writing style that is both entertaining and thought provoking, Dave Draper cuts through all the hype and psuedo-science that dominates the world of fitness today."

—*Bill Keyes, strength coach*

"Simply the best book on training. Bar none. I'll never need another bodybuilding book again."

—*Douglas Malcolm, BookIdeas.com*

"I've been a connoisseur of weight-lifting books for more than 30 years. *Brother Iron, Sister Steel* has encapsulated the useful information from them all in this one inspiring and motivating book."

—*Guy Miller, Performance Operations Manager*

"Solidly affirming... Entertaining, even philosophical. ...fun, informative, and (I have to say it) brawny..."

—*D. Patrick Miller, Fearless Reviews*

"Powerfully good writer... Part exercise strategy, part memoir, part motivational training guide... manages to be highly entertaining on all counts."

—*Tai Moses, Metro Magazine*

"You'll get hooked on *Brother Iron, Sister Steel*. In every word, Draper leaves the mark of his genius."

—*Julian Schmidt, Flex Magazine*

# Your Body Revival

*Weight Loss Straight Talk*

## Dave Draper

On Target Publications - Aptos, California

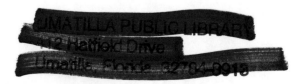

*Your* Body Revival: *Weight Loss Straight Talk*
by Dave Draper

Copyright © 2002 Dave Draper
First Printing August 2002

Also by Dave Draper:
*Brother Iron, Sister Steel: A Bodybuilder's Book*

Published by:
On Target Publications
P. O. Box 1335
Aptos, CA 95001 USA
(888) 466-9185
info@ontargetpublications.com
www.ontargetpublications.com

Cover photo: Elan Sun Star
Foreword: Mike Nichols, M.D.
Copyeditor: Cheryl Stewart-Miller
Cover design: Valarie Howell/Howell Graphics
All unattributed verses and quotes by Dave Draper

Library of Congress Cataloging-in-Publication Data

Draper, Dave.
  Your body revival : weight loss straight talk / Dave Draper.
      p. cm.
Includes bibliographical references and index.
  ISBN 1-931046-35-2
  1. Weight loss. I. Title.
  RM222.2 .D695 2002
  613.7—dc21

                                        2001006376

## Author's Note
## Who am I and where are we going?

The book is completed. The copyeditor has pawed over the pages and did her best to untangle the knots. The cover design is in its final stages and the book is ready to go to print. However, as it is with all projects large and small, two nagging concerns bob at the surface and gain my attention: The reader doesn't know the writer and, perhaps, the writer fails to engage the reader. I worry that I have prepared a soup that no one will eat. It will sit steaming in its bowl and grow cold, neither stirred, sniffed nor sampled.

Who I am is the easy one. Dave Draper, your humble servant and former Mr. New Jersey, Mr. America, Mr. Universe and Mr. World of the '60s and '70s; at the writing of this book, 58 years old and 47 years in the pursuit of fitness. I have stumbled like a dolt on clay feet, which only served to make me stronger. Along with my wife and friends I own and operate two World Gyms on the central coast of California; you can visit my website, IronOnline.com, or read my book on muscle building, *Brother Iron, Sister Steel*, published in January 2001.

My carefully doled-out pride is that I grew up with bodybuilding and physical fitness when it was yet a strong and innocent child, unexploited and unspoiled by modernism—when fact stood apart from fiction and good, old-fashioned hard work was an ethic. I hope to pass these fading qualities on to you.

About engaging the reader? Ah, I quickly take up the spear and shield and go to battle with the determination to win the war against obesity. I fear this solid, bold and mighty approach may wobble the knees of the troops or offend the sensibilities of the modern man. But I'm compelled to rid the dragon of its head, quickly. I call on guts, nerve, toughness and the will to prevail. Are you with me?

If so, I have engaged the reader and together we will win.

Dave Draper
February 2002

# Table of Contents

# Foreword

I have just read the manuscript for the book you now hold in your hands. It is an example of a rare thing: a fine, powerful tool.

Draper's prose is the word equivalent of a clear, steady gaze; authority, experience and honesty stare you dead in the eye. He actually cares whether or not you struggle with being overweight. He actually knows how to help you be more fit than you have ever been in your life. What Dave Draper has discovered in the foundry of his own transformation from shy New Jersey boy to mature and wise bodybuilder is that hard work is ever just that: hard work. Let him take your hand and lead you to that honest workplace where you can begin to be more well and more fit than you have ever been.

As Draper often says, "The secret is there is no secret." While there is no secret, there are many "tricks of the trade." And he knows them all. The truth is, if you know Dave's place in bodybuilding history, you know he is one of the founders of that trade and the author of many of its tricks as well.

I am a physician and know an awful lot of exercise physiology, endocrinology—in fact a whole raft of "ologies"—and still I sit as often as possible at the feet of this master and learn. My knowing cellular energetics and how to activate lipozymes doesn't make the weight any lighter or the miles any shorter. Read this book and learn. Listen to his turns of phrase. They often seem odd, even eccentric, until you discover that they are actually the most concise way to convey the essence of will, of determination, of how to succeed.

My work as a physician is helping people, in as natural a way as possible, to manage their diabetes, their coronary artery disease, and their other diseases often caused by bad habits and the press of time. Obesity is intertwined with this list to a remarkable degree. Thus, this is an important book. It offers a straight shot at solving one of the root causes of most diseases. I mean what that last sentence said; getting control of your body fat does not ensure immortality, but it does substantially decrease the risk of premature death and debility. And this book is just the tool to help you gain that control.

Mike Nichols, M.D.
The Tempus Clinic
Los Gatos, California

# Preface

We live in a miraculous world during turbulent times. I offer a concise book to my fellow world travelers who recognize the existence of urgent problems that need to be examined and fixed. The specific problem with which I am concerned is that of being overweight or, more accurately, over fat. As the title suggests, I address the overweight with no accusation, sense of apology or socially polite verbiage. I allow little slack. There's no time or need for conciliatory language and happy-face tolerance in approaching the dilemma before us. Trifling is, in fact, a large part of the problem.

It's inconceivable that modern man, the designer of the space shuttle, satellite communication, heart transplants and life-extending biotech breakthroughs, is buried with an overweight disaster of epidemic proportions. He's eating his way to death. Amid his busy schedule he has paused and noted that he and his children are getting fatter every day; it is a problem nearing a crisis and needs the world's undivided attention.

I refer to the unhealthy and unfit condition of society as a reflection of its apathy, complacency and unawareness. My references are not insensitive comments on the undesirable fitness level of the people on the streets. They are not condemnations but instructive urgings to set the inactive into motion. They are not intended to ridicule the overweight but, rather, to stir the dozing. They call the weak to strength with no tone of mocking in the voice. The mocking, rather, is in the ear.

Exercising regularly and eating smartly prepare us for the tough days ahead. Exercise is a constructive diversion that relaxes and reduces stress; strengthens the body, mind and spirit; establishes confidence; builds brother- and sisterhood; adds considerably to the resources of the country and prepares it to win the good fight.

I'm concerned, curious and excited. Years gone by have demonstrated that the process of untangling ourselves from crises renders us a marvelous creature. Examining and resolving obesity will generate a smarter and more grateful mankind, enriching our days. I'm an optimist.

Let's apply the proper words to define our physical potential—solid, bold and mighty.

There's only one way to lose weight wisely and permanently, and it's no secret. It's simple, but it's not easy: exercise and eat right, consistently. My hope and mission is to persuade you to follow the only way, the seemingly bleak way, with joy and conviction. Let's transform black and white into color, the clank of metal into music and the craving for junk food into a hunger for personal growth. What daily activities are more basic and natural, more productive and fulfilling than attending our health, happiness and long life?

Ready… on your mark… get set…

# Chapter 1

## Your Body Revival:
### *Weight Loss Straight Talk*

It appears that losing weight has become one of mankind's social pastimes, a big industry for the resourceful businessperson and a specialty in the medical community. Motivation for the overweight and plans to follow in the quest for trimness are the subjects of numerous books, magazines, clubs, clinics and commercial weight-loss centers around the world. There are neighborhood programs and online support groups that point the anxious and needy in the right direction, but they serve more as a crutch than a fix. I could dig in and present a string of suggestions on why and how to lose weight with psychological underpinnings, but will they penetrate, provoke and stimulate? Even the optimist in me thinks probably not. Will the ordinary words, the ever-loving clichés rephrased grab hold and shake the hungry and dismayed reader into action, or will they evaporate like steam from a boiling kettle?

Not wanting to exercise the involuntary reflex of pitching a "sure-fire" weight-loss program, I have prepared a heartfelt, long-overdue, point-blank approach that I believe can do no worse.

It goes something like this...

My name is Dave Draper and I'm your friend. What I am about to say is harsh and disturbing—it is meant to be—but in no way is it designed to violate or demean you, the reader. We are, in spite of all our strengths, proliferated with weakness. Let the strong rally and wrestle to the Earth's rugged surface a fair share of those limitations and set a high mark for the less brave that surround us.

The masses of the modern world are getting fatter and less fit every day, an inexcusable combination that profiles man's deteriorating backbone, character and instincts. Where we were once hardy, square-shouldered and erect, we are now stooped and burdened. Where once we ran and played, we now stumble and grope.

The precious fresh fruits, vegetables and hearty proteins that nourish our bodies have lost their appeal and been replaced by sugar, fat and chemicals in a bag, to go.

Like sheep gone astray, we are accompanying one another to the slaughter: dumb, fat, lazy and meek. It doesn't stop there. We know better and we ignore the dilemma. We deny and we procrastinate. We avoid considering the eventual consequences of our over-consuming as if by magic they might not one day visit us, personally. Stroke, heart attack, diabetes, shortness of breath? Oh, no, thanks, I gave at the office. Maybe next year. We find comfort in the overwhelming presence of others of similar structure and countenance and convince ourselves of the normalcy of corpulence. The descriptive word "fat" is no longer a socially correct term and we shy of its use should we offend the deceived ego and start a war. Veiled eyes dart to another distraction (TV, video games, obsessive work, food, drink) and the pain of reality is quieted again.

My harshness is kindness in disguise. Does one tell a child about to thrust his hand into the beehive to enjoy the honey?

We can fix the problem. You who dare read this verbal affront to self-destruction—one's continued contribution to a fattened and deteriorating body—are only a nod from the solution. Stop here for a moment and consider the common crossroads before you.

Each road, at first sight, is similar in appearance and takes you along your way in everyday travel. One, a common road, goes left and abruptly downhill with no margins on the food you eat, no exercise, no real disciplines, no hope. Discarded fast-food bags, Big Gulps and beer cans litter the muddy ditches and blinking neon—Eat 'n' Go—illuminates the brooding, overcast sky. The other road bends to the right with a gradual uphill grade that wanders through tilled farmland, orchards and meadows of grazing cattle. It's called the high road where the air is fresh, the water is pure and good eating habits are shared generously. Exciting workouts charge the body and there's a gym just over the hill and another in a warm, sunny valley.

Do you want to be among the fat and the lazy? Is that a self-image you are willing to accept? Do you like to be out of control? Are you content being one of the mindless masses, the ordinary on their way down the wrong road? Don't be offended, deny, rationalize or blame. You have passions and opinions; you protect your rights and options and you're a good person with intelligence and aspiration. Furthermore, you have arms and legs and a will. Why not apply these qualities to the preservation of your life? Gather them together, multiply them like earnings and enhance your days.

Your choice, your decision: left or right?

What difference does it make which way I should go? Why, if not asked to pause, I would surely go slightly downhill as it appears to be easier and, by evidence of its broadness and trodden surface, it is the road most traveled, probably safer. That's for me: easier and safer.

Think twice. Easier and safer leads to rounder and softer amid a crowd of the dull-eyed. Go right and feel the wind, the flexing of your muscles and, ah… hear the sound of music, one sure step at a time, day after glorious day. There's a perceptible difference—an appealing difference—in the effort of travel and soon you define it as stimulating and invigorating, a fulfilling adventure without which you would despair.

The choice, to be effective and comprehensive, needs to originate in the center of your being where hope resides. Only when you review your nature and are dismayed by its composition, only when you are struck with purpose, impelled by its power and visualize transformation, will you raise your head and say, "I'm going right; I'm taking the high road, where life is lived and honored and cherished."

Somewhere along our journey we have forgotten our responsibility—our obligation—to care for our body and maintain its well-being. Respect for the fragile and intricate vehicle in which we travel is seldom considered. The least we can do is feed it nourishing food and gratefully, lovingly nurture it with exercise. There are rare exceptions, and I suspect you and I are listed among them, but the majority are ignorant, just along for the ride till the ride gives out.

## No one stands above the fight

I'm careful not to judge, ridicule or condescend, yet the message I choose to relate is hard and must be driven home hard. What good is it if the facts and figures are offered with euphemisms and mildness as the intended recipients are stroked and lulled and treated as if fatness is a common dilemma we should one day address?

It is not unlikely in some instances that obesity is the symptom of a sickness of far greater significance than poor body composition and an overtaxed system. Consider apathy, the boundless spirit tethered, calmed to complacency, and void of motivation, aspiration and interest. It's not hopelessness; it's never having hoped. Exercise and diet? Not now; tomorrow, perhaps. Pass the potato chips and remote control, please.

Only with you fully on my side can we confront the topic before us. I have spoken candidly about the ever-growing condition of modern man's waistline. The subject is serious and delicate and, therefore, difficult to approach. How do I speak of man's fatness without hurting, angering or demeaning the beholder while none of these notions are intended? I pause, write, delete and pause again.

Are you still with me? I'm somewhere between 50 and 100 and not without my loss of years. Though I've never let go of hard exercise and right eating, I romped in bad habits long enough to crash. Thus, as I take aim at mankind and ask where his sense of responsibility has gone or remind him of the gift of life, I am not without being wounded by my own words. It's your obligation, I shout, to care for your body, mind and soul, and I submerge in bittersweet humiliation. I have made the mistakes. The time I lost has been my gain; I'm wiser and able to tell you.

Take hold of your life with thanksgiving.

# Chapter 2

## Something's Happening Here:
### *Obesity Statistics & Trends*

I was told by an outstanding novelist at a local book signing that the job of a writer is to engage the reader's attention with the opening sentence and carry him through the pages as if on a magic carpet... or something like that. Chapter two and already I have a problem and need your help. Does this follow the technique recommended by my friend, the novelist, or does this shake your confidence in me, who has done nothing yet to gain it? Let me explain.

The theme of *Your Body Revival* occurred to me a year ago and is developing as I write. My intention is to approach those burdened with extra body fat and all its encumbrances with a firm tone and unwavering eyes. I dare you to face the truth of obesity with me by your side, and I promise to help you resolve your dilemma with courage and might.

And so, the story unfolds, the pages emerge from the printer and the message digs into the envisioned reader's mind. I sit back and read the first dozen pages. Tough words and they grab the problem from every angle, reveal it, shake it, magnify it and flood it with uncompromising light. Part one of my mission is complete—exposure of the raw, unforgiving, unforgivable overweight condition. Things are looking mighty grim for the reader. Hmm. Exactly what I intended, but I'm beginning to feel like a creep, dirty rat... a scruffy, flea-bitten hound dawg.

Phase two of my inspiring plan is to place my arm around you, the reader, and assure you of my understanding and knowledge and my compassion for your plight. "Yes, I know your life is not midnight black and hope is in your every breath, but I have walked the less-beaten path and I entreat you to follow." Vaguely arrogant and it's a rub, but I must gain your trust.

I'm on schedule, the grisly subject matter is on paper and I'm satisfied. Briefly. I recall my writer friend and his entreaty to engage the reader and carry him on a magic carpet ride. Ha. Magic carpet? This is more like a worn-out welcome mat tumbling through Hurricane Hugo. Who is going to read my ranting and raving for two pages, never mind 10? I won't engage them; I'll enrage them. No one will read past the first diatribe that roars from the flamethrower that is my blistered mind without tossing the darn book out the window. I'm feeling alone with my words.

Over 250 pages of information, stories and encouragement will sit in the cold, still darkness of a closed volume dedicated to truth and freedom. Will the good reader, for whose favor I plead and whose attention I am jealous, continue to turn the pages? Will he read my solutions, my pitch for good health and lost weight, strong muscles and a shapely form? Only if I beg. What must I do to breach the ragged gap that honesty stripped bare of subtlety creates, the pain of bleak reality exposed? Beg…on hands and knees… beseech…

A plea: Please, read the first couple dozen pages as a writ of passage, and hang onto the promising words that follow. They will lead you to honest weight loss and a healthful, long life. No good thing is free.

## Get outta town

My wife, Laree, and I enjoy taking off in the car and heading across the country. Between projects when the time and the season are right, we'll pick a spot on the map and go. There's freedom in the open road, and pulling off the interstate in the middle of nowhere is always an adventure. Not exactly tracking grizzly in the northwest Rockies, but, hey, I'm from Jersey, right? Besides, eating at a convenient off-ramp restaurant can be almost as hair raising.

Hungry and wiggly only a day into our most recent cruise, we coasted down an exit and ground to a halt at the first promising café amid a small city of fast-food eateries. The sign in the window said something about home cooking. Yeah, right. We managed to manipulate the menu to provide all the protein, carbs and fats we needed, and sat back to absorb the surroundings. It was during this trip, a lazy drive to spacious Colorado, that I decided to write this book.

Our power meal was served with little confusion; Laree and I sat back to eat and observe. People watching. Anybody can do it—I did it on my first try. The rules are simple. You must not judge, mock or condescend. However, emotions are the underpinning of free-spirited highway travelers. We did our best.

A family of four walked slowly in our direction and climbed into the booth next to us. They looked tired—like it was a long hike from the front counter, but they made it. The dad was a gentle guy who, after brief negotiations, ordered the food. Mom fussed in her backpack and passed out what appeared to be recently snapped photos of the kids, a girl and a boy in their middle teens. Comments were made; reactions and smiles filled the table. They were good people and, when the food came, I was disturbed and saddened, but not surprised. What I observed was typical and where the sweet family was headed was predictable. They were silent while they devoured their extra-large portions of pasta, pizza, burgers, fries and coke. They ordered dessert and I tried not to look.

We paid our bill, and on the way out felt as if we were escaping. The parents were not yet 40, retaining remnants of attractive youth and 30 extra pounds each. The kids were shy and cute and innocent and held 50 too many pounds between them. I believe they all knew it, and I wanted to cry, especially for the cute young girl.

There grew a discomfort within me that I couldn't define. I was happy, yet discouraged. Life, rollercoaster that it is, was good, yet I was depressed. I strive to be positive amid the fray and seldom fail. What was wrong?

The lengthening spring evening was ahead and we were on a gentle rise well out of town, the sprawl behind us. Leaning against the hood of the vehicle with crossed arms, I scanned the desperate oasis surrounding me. Three gas station quick-stops and a dozen fast-food joints refueling the thirsty vehicles and their hungry passengers stood out amid the mild rolling hills.

"Laree, are we alone here? Does anyone know how much junk they're eating?" Always determined that my questions not go unanswered, she suggested we take a tour of the thriving environs. The night was young. We were ever hopeful.

We walked into establishment number-one for a peek. Astonishing. Everyone was eating with two fists and talking at the same time. Those who moved about displayed large midsections and little muscle in the arms. Bad combination.

Establishment number-two had a frenzied food-to-go window and the consumers were patient and mostly round. They drank jumbo colas and smiled as they waited. The glitzy, snappy, all-glass third enterprise had the children's attention. Kids played hi-tech arcade games as the parents battled the front lines. Lots of fries 'n' chili dogs a foot long and candied chicken wings in this neighborhood. I must have said "Yuck" out loud because everyone turned and Laree jabbed me in the ribs. We hit the road.

Our fast-food excursion that night was fortifying as we didn't eat a thing, nor were we tempted, and we felt like Olympic athletes. It was also enlightening. We'd been ensconced in our World Gym on the California coast for10 years and forgot what people outside our neck of the woods ate and looked like.

The night closed in around us as we motored on and emptied another tank of gas. Time for another roadside adventure to include the supermarket and a motel where the sign read "Vacancy." Reviewing our day and planning the next kept us busy until we lit the fuse to the nefarious TV. The news was frightening and the commercials mouth watering. We sat in bed and grew sleepy watching the fast-food sponsors compete for our appetites between 10-minute glimpses of a Bogart-Bacall classic. Last thing I remember Humphrey B. was ordering a SuperMac and fries for two.

Early the next morning, bright-eyed and trim but not smug (doesn't take much for either one of us to feel dumpy), we resumed our cross-country trek. The miles zoomed by and we talked about our curious response to the neon-flickering beehive of fat, sugar and lost control. The diversion we had originally planned started to take on another form. I found myself loving life yet distressed that my brothers and sisters were engaged in what appeared to be unsuspecting self-destruction. The killer is not the definite evils of smoking or booze or drugs. It's Happy Jack's food in the two-for-one jumbo sizes, and its killing effect is a hundred times subtler but just as deadly. I started to keep mental notes of the human condition now distinct in my mind. The eating habits, the fat size and the lack of muscle tone; and the attitude, appearance and the countenance of the men, women, boys and girls around me became my general focus. How snoopy can you get? Laree joined in.

I repeatedly assured myself that these were well-intentioned observations to assist in compiling material for a book for the overweight, the book you are now reading. The time was enjoyably spent, as work and play have always defined my life. (The gyms we own are, after all, giant toy boxes, and gym owners will often comment that owning a gym sure beats working for a living.)

The following day I began a survey that had structure.

Exercising my eagle eye and uncanny ability to evaluate the human anatomy at a glance, I mentally documented the number of people who were overweight. I categorized them by gender, age range and estimated over-fat category (over 30 pounds and over 60 pounds). Do this for a day or two and you sketch a general representation and gain a broad sense of the problem.

I'm a master sleuth. Here's my report: Six out of 10 are at least 30 pounds overweight (considered obese) and, of those, three are 60 pounds over the acceptable mark. Big. One out of 20 had a middle girth that exceeded any norm I had witnessed before. Really big. I was shocked to notice that today's standard for a large belly protudes five inches more than it did last time I wandered the surface of the earth five years ago. Surprisingly, if this was a contest between the men and the women, it would be a tie. The kids followed their parents but had not yet caught up. Five out of 10 needed to play more and eat less. Teen girls were having a tougher time staying trim. Guys can pretend it's bulky muscle and wear an over-sized Raider's jacket; most girls prefer hip-huggers. Other indicators—eyes, expressions, mannerisms, displayed mentality, dress, walk and energy—were observed by my nosey glances and served to guide me in subtler ways.

## The big picture few see

We're slipping, and I'm troubled. We've strayed from healthy physical activity and have served up for ourselves a lifestyle of distractions from reality and oversized platters of greasy and sugary food. Certain I am not assuming a superior or judgmental position, I declare alarm for many of those around me. The majority of the folks across the land are soft, unconditioned and vulnerable. My emotional responses had an interesting order: at first, disappointment, quickly to be replaced by sadness mixed with compassion; anger was aroused at some point when irresponsibility was clearly reflected; and, finally, the fear of our weakness as a society loomed above the rest. The overweight condition is frightening.

I'm not a crusader and I don't envision myself fighting crime or the larger wrongs of the world. They're not acceptable, but they're inevitable. I leave them to the experts and authorities. However, in the battle against the wrong we do to ourselves physically on a daily basis, I take up arms. This is individual, personal and controllable. It's not illogical to say that to the degree that we neglect our health and fitness, we neglect one another. Take a close look. Beware lest we become weak; prone to illness, disease and injury; easy prey to resistance; ineffective and apathetic.

It's a matter of personal and national security to exercise and eat right for good. We depend on one another.

What shall we do?

Read on with confidence and commitment. The expanded version, outlined in the pages ahead, underscores the immediate need for the overweight to start moving. Action now. It helps to understand an adversary completely before we can wrestle it to the ground. We dig into the overeating issues. The foods we eat are examined, and we determine a food plan to vitalize the body and claim a healthy weight. Exercise is brought boldly to the foreground and we begin to build muscle and might.

You've probably heard it all before. We could spend the day together going through the local library and discover at least a hundred volumes dedicated to diet and weight loss. There is no shortage of good and bad information, ideas and fads in the written word. I'm quick to point out that the day would be better spent lifting weights at the gym and eating protein, but sufficient review and organized thought is essential; there's a place for the written word.

My purpose is to stimulate, motivate, encourage, harass, pressure, caution and compel you to take the right steps in the right direction. The necessary facts are here in this volume as I see them and as I've lived them. My successes and errors and those I've observed in the world around me are evident in the pages ahead. Nothing earthshaking; just simple truths.

Were the words that follow spread before you as a fabric, they would not be a fine silk cloth, but more closely resemble a rough tapestry of reclaimed threads, a broad weave of experience and expression to clothe you from head to toe.

As a lifter I've never been overweight, though fat seems to haunt everyone I know, even the skinny. That obesity and poor conditioning are severe afflictions has become plain and clear to me through my years in the gym as a user and owner. I fight fat daily as I seek muscle and power. I prescribe regular weight training, sound eating and smart living to our gym members to achieve a healthy body weight and total fitness.

Life's a journey, full of detours and washed-out bridges. I'll help you overcome them— I promise—though sometimes I can be a nuisance. Throughout your travels to change your weight, strength and health, you'll be changing your life. Does change sound frightening? Getting stronger every day in every way is exhilarating. It grows on you and that, too, I promise.

# Chapter 3

## Who are You & Where are You Going?
### *Goals & Possibilities*

Let's get underway, right here, right now. As I continue to mix mortar and lay stones, consider this chapter the start of your application to lose the weight. I offer you in morsels the untangled information to get you where you want to go. This is founded on basic truths that we'll ruminate, observations of others with similar targets, interviews and surveys that I personally initiated, conferences with dedicated professionals and, finally, my own "Johnny-on-the-Spot" experiences— nothing like real life to teach you a thing or two.

I'm not convinced a lot of technical information and detailed research will win the war; fascinating fodder for strategists but not for us gritty soldiers in the trenches. We've got battles to win day after day. Action—That's how victory is gained. I've watched and listened to people who read, write, study and attend seminars and then achieve nothing in the way of weight loss, muscle gain or health. They are prepared to lecture on the subjects but apply none of the principals they studied, as if knowing the problem was enough. Application of knowledge—not knowledge itself—brings forth change.

And now, ladies and gentlemen, I present to you the star of the show, the amazing, the fantastic, the one and only… at this point I introduce you and you step forward, bow humbly, yet surely, and tell us who you are, where you are going. Take your time because the story begins here.

You need to look at yourself, starting with the exterior and penetrating to the interior where your thinking occurs and your feelings arise freely. This isn't a casual glance—name, age, gender, hair color, height and weight. This is a sensible, comprehensive examination. Do you want to know where you're going? You need to know who you are.

Know thyself. Sit, think, meditate about yourself and get comfortable doing it. *Your Body Revival* does not engage in touchy-feely techniques, self-help passivity or I-love-me-I-deserve-it activity. Okay? I encourage a healthy introspection to get you familiar with your strengths, weaknesses and peculiarities: to see them clearly and laugh, admire, appreciate and apply them or eradicate them. I prompt you to do this because it works to confront your desire to lose weight, and because we generally avoid constructive self-evaluation. We often bring forth our weaknesses to brood over and punish ourselves. We polish our strengths to brighten our ego and raise our conceit. No, not this bright and sunny point in time. Today, you identify who you are, honestly, and engineer in the days to come the best-made plan for you to lose weight and be strong.

It's easy. I notice that I am selfish down to the bone, mean, unscrupulous and troublesome. So, I'm ordinary. Recognize the face in your mental mirror before you make plans to improve it. This exercise can be practiced whenever you realize its value, feel comfortable and have the urge. It's something we do silently all day long—isn't it?—though I call for a constructive and conscious effort. Have fun.

What characteristic about you might prevent you from succeeding?

As I look out over the faces, I think I recognize a few. You've been around awhile, are on fairly safe ground and need only to lose a few pounds and stick with the program. You need a nudge to get you going, a shot of reassurance that you're not alone and a convincing reminder that getting fit is exceedingly important. You need a review of the basics, the truths by which we live. Not many, but a handful, are only pounds and inches away from being toned and you hope there's something in these pages that you've overlooked and which will jump out at you. I wouldn't be surprised. By golly, neighbors, Engineer Dave is here to put you back on track and convince you that any other train is an express to disappointment on down the line. As they say over at Grand Central, "My train or the mule train."

We're often alone and need to be tough each and every day of our lives. I know the road is narrow and cruel for some whose abilities are limited, and I know also that eating disorders are bandits along the way. Anorexia nervosa, bulimia and binging are beyond my scope, but not beyond my concern. Depression is a millstone that can be unloosed. I know there is hope in these pages if there is hope in you, if there is hope in me. Turn the pages one by one and read the jumbled text. It's not unusual that among the thorns a flower grows, a common thought rephrased or a word repeated at the right time strikes your mind and inspiration floods the body and spirit.

Exhilarating.

## Tarnished goals in their splendor

Goals are a wonderful thing. They exist in the background of our mind and subtly move us along the corridors of life. This grand feature of the psyche has been observed by doctors of the mind and they have encouraged us to define our goals to shape our lives. By them we might very well define our future, step forward, remain in place or devour ourselves in frustration. Conscious and unconscious goals create presidents and champions, criminals and saints. They get us up in the morning and off to school, work and play. Sometimes it's a small, yet significant, goal that keeps us alive from morning to evening, day after day. And, goals have substance, yet only to the degree that we believe in them and reach for them with all our heart's energy. Our desire.

Don't underestimate the power of goal setting or overestimate the goal you set. Foolish goals can have us crawling across the Sahara without water or seeking solitude in the heart of raging Times Square; they can be dangerous or impossible. What do you want, when, how and why? More specifically, what do you want to weigh and when? What are your diet plans, exercise plans and motivations? What frustrates you? Fair considerations, don't you agree?

Here's a list of inquiries to ponder before writing down your goals in indelible ink. I ran a similar survey in the spring of 2001 before

5,000 IronOnline.com email newsletter readers. One hundred-fifty brave souls responded in detail. They all agreed that answering the questions helped them to know themselves—sound familiar?—and was an important exercise in their ongoing challenge to lose weight and get fit. The insight gained from the e-interview has been liberally applied to these pages.

Relax. We are simply familiarizing, digging around our own back-yards and turning over a few stones in the gardens. Sufficient self-evaluation never hurts, always helps. I'll caution you periodically not to be overly self-critical as it's certain to give you a stiff neck. Reference points, however, will be helpful. If you find yourself nodding off or wiggling in your seat, move on. None of us will think of you as lazy or cowardly.

We'll work on diet and exercise together, soon. Smart eating and vigorous training are a joy waiting breathlessly in the wings.

Quick thoughts: Read through the list entirely to review the questions and grasp their concepts. Return to answer the questions and you'll find them less daunting and your answers more comprehensive and meaningful.

## Eighteen root questions

**1.** Approximately how many pounds overweight are you?

**2.** When did you realize it was a problem, distraction or distress? How long have you actively sought weight loss and fitness? Have you previously tested your resolve through fad diets and exercise programs?

**3.** What do you consider the contributing factors to your overweightness: pregnancy, illness, injury, overwork or life's busy paths? Psychological predisposition, definable eating disorder? Genetics?

**4.** What steps have you taken—consistently or inconsistently—to overcome the situation?

**a.** Diets: History specifics—high protein-low carbohydrate, vegetarian, low fat-high carbohydrate, starvation diet, Atkins, Pritikin, cabbage, ketogenic. Were they significant efforts for considerable time? Hit and miss, yo-yo? Did any work well or appear to have promise?

**b.** Exercise: History specifics—walk, jog, resistence exercise, sports, aerobics, dance. How long and what level of input?

**5.** Consider your medical history: Have you seen a doctor recently for a physical evaluation? Heart health, blood pressure, hyper- or hypo-glycemia, thyroid or hormonal dysfunction—medications prescribed. No? Make an appointment. Other professional care (personal trainer, dietitian, alternative medicine, hypnosis, voodoo)?

**6.** Is your particular overweight condition a complex medical problem involving systemic or chemistry disorder? Treatable? There are medical conditions that are chronic or of a severe nature that apparently deny remedy. Don't give up.

**7.** Review your vast storehouse of character traits and inner fiber: discipline, focus, resolve, patience, perseverance, hopefulness and commitment. Do you shine as brightly as the morning sun or are you illuminated by the light of the new moon? We will fix these things, you and I. Add trust to the above list.

**8.** What is your current state of mind: relaxed or anxious? Is your attitude positive or negative? Are you comfortable with yourself, confident, generally happy or sad, insecure, angry, moody, docile or aggressive?

Humor me... I'm writing a book.

**9.** Analyze your current lifestyle. Do you relax at home, or do you party or eat out often? Do you get enough sleep? Are you willing to alter any habits that will slow down your fat-loss progress or would you rather make goals that will allow more tolerance in your lifestyle?

Hey, you okay? You look a little bewildered. Take five. This can be an exhausting exercise in itself. Unless these questions were prepared and proposed by someone else, it is doubtful you would concoct them and answer them like a clown. This is more fun than a mirror when you least expect it. Keep going; you're the greatest.

**10.** Note your occupational demands (stress, overtime, 9 to 5, physically tough, corporate pressure, doctor, lawyer, Indian chief). How much time is available to dedicate to training each week? Can you and are you willing to schedule meal breaks?

**11.** Has motivation been an underlying problem with correcting your body composition? Do you care enough to try hard enough to bring balance to your system?

**12.** Are lack of discipline and commitment preventing you from proceeding on an intelligent plan to resolve your problem? Do thoughts of exercise and diet make you depressed, nervous and irritable? Do they stir excitement?

**13.** Are you confused by the abundance of mixed information about health and weight loss?

**14.** What holds you back? Lack of fortitude, no support, apathetic, demoralized, defeated... I'm lazy, who cares? Why bother? It's too late. Maybe you're not tough enough or your weight's such a common problem that you feel quite normal and almost comfortable.

**15.** Obvious question: What are your current nutritional habits and what were they in your earlier years? Do you enjoy good, wholesome food or do you need fast foods or sweets to satisfy your appetite? How do you rate your appetite control level, with one representing the pits and 9.9 the peaks?

**16.** Are you planning to exercise? Where? Home, local gym or a question mark? Are you comfortable at the gym? Is it adequate, frilly, clubby or next to the boiler room in the crumbling YMCA? This is important; don't make any further membership arrangements until you complete *Your Body Revival*. Okay?

**17.** Are you alone in your quest or do you have a partner you can count on? Is your partner committed to the same goals? Work on this list together. Very revealing, and revelation is a step to salvation.

**18.** This is not a sales gimmick: Were you absolutely convinced there was a right plan for you, would you follow it with diligence and confidence to realize its merits? Hardly, totally, partially, probably not? The question is a test of skepticism and commitment. Some doubt there is a scheme that will work for them and others will hardly try if there is. Your initial reaction to the question is probably your answer.

## Are you serious? Goals anyone?

Man, by nature, is a goal-oriented creature and goal setting has become more than a primal function. Imagery and visualizing (using our imagination to maximize our aspirations) have become effective and practical in business, sports and medicine. "I can if I think I can," and "I'm getting better every day in every way" are axioms that seem to work in today's pressing world. "I'm a big, bad, muscle machine" has always been one of my favorites.

High school reminder: Goal setting is the number-one key to weight-loss success and can be divided into two basic categories: long-term goals, what you expect to achieve in the years to come, and short-term goals, what you expect to achieve in the next days and weeks. Make no mistake: These need to be addressed thoughtfully to ensure clear and positive action.

It is time for you to polish your goals like golden apples and list them for everyone, especially you, to see. Referencing past experiences and observations and the new ones brought to light in reading *Your Body Revival*, where are you heading? What image do you have of yourself? In what time frame are you working? By what means do you intend to accomplish your goals? How much are you willing to compromise?

Pad and pen ready? You have as much time as you need. No cheating.

## Stumbling blocks to surmount

One evening before putting the pen to the page, I created a list of stumbling blocks you might encounter in your struggle to lose fat and get in shape. The following nouns, verbs, adjectives and descriptive phrases are intended to ring a bell and remind you of the unstable territory you are about to cross—a little warm-up to stimulate the appropriate juices and nudge the sometime-dormant senses to consciousness as you set out to conquer the foe, obesity.

Incidentally, I use the words obesity, overweight, large, heavy and fat interchangeably to mean the same physical state: carrying excessive body mass in the form of fat.

Cheer up. Almost certainly 10 of the following transgressions are not on your list and five can be eliminated before the day's end. Some, however, like putting bears in a cage, will be very resistant.

1. *Smoking*
2. *Drinking, drugs*
3. *Partying*
4. *Junk food... chips and dip, cottton candy and Ritz crackers*
5. *Fast food... McD and the gang*
6. *Snacking... anything, any ole' time*
7. *Sugar... sugar and more sugar*
8. *Lack of exercise*
9. *Couch potato—general inactivity*
10. *Ignorance of the seriousness of being unconditioned and overweight*
11. *Denial... defensiveness*
12. *Aware of the problem but unmotivated*
13. *Not taking action with a responsible exercise plan*
14. *Not showing initiative with a smart nutritional plan*
15. *Undisciplined... disorderly, unorganized, cluttered*
16. *Lazy*
17. *Gluttonous*
18. *Emotional eating: distraction, boredom, reward, eating disorder*
19. *Procrastination*
20. *Hopelessness*
21. *Complacency*
22. *Fat and fearful... resistant, unwilling, insecure*
23. *No time... family and job-bound*
24. *Weak-willed*
25. *Lack of support, alone, no one cares*
26. *Don't know where to start, ignorant,  confused*
27. *Yo-yo performer, repeat failure, fear of failing, fad-diet junkie*
28. *Chemistry and genetics*
29. *Quick-fix mentality*
30. *Creature of bad habits: nutritional, exercise, work, lifestyle*

There are a number of hair triggers in this keg of dynamite. Handle with care.

How is your list of goals (a.k.a. imaginings, visions, targets, hopes, wants, needs and desires) coming along?

## 25 common trouble spots for weight-loss participants:

- Health and nutrition are not considered, only weight loss.
- They eat too little and they eat poorly.
- They often starve themselves.
- They eat too infrequently.
- They count calories only, forgoing food balance.
- They eat too little protein.
- They fail to drink enough water.
- They switch weight-loss programs with trends... anxious and immature.
- They cave in to cravings; they leap before looking.
- They give up too soon; they lack commitment.
- They flounder and submit... lack drive.
- They are impatient... childish.
- They are inconsistent... impulsive.
- They don't continue a smart plan once they achieve a degree of success... lack perseverance.
- They don't exercise, hardly exercise or exercise too mildly.
- They don't recognize the importance of muscle presence.
- They exercise the heart, lungs and pulmonary system only.
- They don't exercise to build muscle; they're uninformed.
- They exercise to burn calories only; they're confused.
- They seldom think; they follow.
- Those who think tend to think too much; they intellectualize, over-analyze.
- Those who have underlying psychological problems fail to persist—push past the barriers—with the basic tenants of weight loss that ensure measurable success.
- They often lack courage... internal fortitude and stamina.
- They might be weak-willed, without physical motivation, purpose and aspiration.
- They don't truly consider the consequences of being out of shape; they're sleeping.

# Chapter 4

## The Key—Start Moving:
### *Exercise Now*

A tightrope separates thinking from doing. Thinking, reading and writing balance you atop the precarious thin line, and I plan to excite you into action before we finish this chapter. You are big boys and girls and know that diet and exercise, call them what you will, are the rascals with which you must contend. Today you start walking, one step at a time across the great divide. Last week I read a couple of popular books for overweight "Dummies" and "Idiots" (strangers to us, obviously) and the authors suggested that part of the exercise plan for couch-ridden dieters includes hiding the remote for the television. This clever trick causes you to stand up from the comfy couch, walk two steps to the tube, change channels, walk two steps back to the comfy couch and sit; repeat when changing the volume. A bit extreme—you might want to pack a lunch—but the author does point out in 25 words or less the importance of exercise.

Exercise rules; it is king of the hill, commander in chief, captain of the ship, head honcho and big mama. Start exercising in a basic and functional way. Think of it as a mild practice, a gesture to molify the silly author (moï), a curious appraisal of "you vs. activity" or a casual nudge of thy roundish flesh-and-bone to get it rolling. Nice and easy does it. Of course, you just might be entrenched in training and fully armed; before you I stand and respectfully bow. Or, perhaps, you cannot wait to break into that once-familiar, old-time feeling where the miles slip behind you and the iron melts in your hands. Routines and schemes I have for the timid and the eager.

As I always say, "This is what I would do if I were you,"—the only pretext under which I dare to advise.

Today, now, in fact, remove the wing tips, high heels or galoshes and replace them with your favorite sneakers. Here is why they call them sneakers: Nonchalant, you step out the front door, acknowledge the world and, as if in a secret disguise, start walking... mildly, at first. Whistle in case anyone is looking (yourself included) and misinterprets your act as exercise. Walking is an amazing form of transportation and gets us where we are going. Running, when possible, is faster. You up to it? Walk for three minutes and jog (your favorite version) for 15 seconds, then walk for a minute and jog 15 seconds. Perform the latter segment (walk and jog) six times and walk home for the next three minutes or so. You've accumulated about 15 minutes of action and probably covered an enviable mini-mile. You are rolling.

Do you feel warm all over and a trickle of water running down your temple and forehead? That's good, old-fashioned, hard-earned, ever-loving perspiration reminding us to drink water, lots of pure water. Water is our friend.

Don't stop now. Let's maintain the heart rate, the body heat and that satisfying feeling. You've got five minutes... let's work the abdominal area, or as I prefer to call it, the midsection. Lie down on your back on a stretch of rug that bears your name. Cradle your head in your hands, bend your knees and draw your feet in tight to stabilize your body. Now, with your feet still on the floor, roll up by the contraction of your abdominal muscles into a "C" position. Exhale during the action, contract tightly, then inhale as you return slowly to the starting position. You're crunching, grasshopper. Repeat this terrific movement for a total of 15 repetitions.

Moving right along, with outstretched arms place your palms downward and under your tailbone. You are about to perform good, old-fashioned floor leg raises. Yes! Bend your knees slightly (or a lot, to diminish resistance) and raise your feet and legs to a near-overhead position, pause and return to the floor. Exhale as you exert on the upward movement and inhale as you lower your legs to the starting point. Breathing comes naturally and easily the less we think about it.

Count a total of 10 reps (as always, do your best) to complete your set of leg raises. Sit upright to pause for 60 seconds as you do a favorite floor stretch, look around in amazement and recuperate. Repeat this combination again (crunches followed by leg raises), sip some water and you are done for day one.

Do you see what's happening here? You're exercising. The dark cloud that settles over your head day and night is scattering. A rosy light is shining through and you feel mellow. Those of us who work out regularly are excited because we know how close you are to becoming attached to this unlikely, cold and clanky, wonderful activity. If only they stick long enough to discover the meaning, we confide, they'll make room for it in their lives, as they do eating, sleeping and working. We know the worth and hidden treasures. We want to share these with you.

Plan to continue the routine described above and work it into your daily schedule. If some days you ache, you'll find a mild warm-up allows you to perform at a comfortable level until you're conditioned and advances can be made. You'll be bugging me about your next workout any day now. As my grandpa used to say when I was a little fella no bigger than a flea, "Son, ya gotta grow roots before ya can grow apples."

Trailing thoughts: Laree just came back from a walk down a steep hill through the redwoods and back again. It took her 10 minutes; she walks it daily and finds it friendly and stimulating. She confesses that it's an easy adjunct to her gym training and extending it might improve its effectiveness. She is also quick to point out that extending the walk might cause her to greet it less enthusiastically and, perhaps, eliminate it all together.

Get up. Get going. Be gone.

# Walk & Jog
*First stages of exercise*

Planning to exercise is often more grueling than actually doing it. I have long admired the famous axiom, "just do it," and I have outlined a simple training approach to accomplish exactly that. Step out your front door and go.

Walk for five minutes.

Immediately, I need to preface my recommendations. Practice the outline below, intending to make modifications according to your physical condition and resolve. I like the mild energy and appeal of the walk and jog combination that follows.

Walk for five minutes—jog for 15 seconds
Walk for one minute—jog for 15 seconds
Walk for one minute—jog for 15 seconds

Repeat the above three combinations for a total of six times.

Walk the remainder of the designated 15 minutes or one mile; your choice.

You're home. Now, you might consider the crunches and leg raises for five minutes.

Thinking of alterations, experiment with increasing the jog time and decreasing the walk time over succeeding workouts. Adding distance or time or days effectively customizes the routine.

Reminders: Take your time to condition yourself and don't chase away your enthusiasm with the old "more is better" credo. Padded Mother Earth is better than concrete—less impact and structural stress. Good sneakers give you comfort and long-lasting running life. Also, you might bring water next time.

# Chapter 5

## Computer Update:
### *Things of the mind*

It's no shocking revelation that the overweight condition is often more complicated than simply carrying excess fat on the body. Many of the problems may very well originate in the mind. It might be the perception one has of oneself that causes obesity or the perception one acquires upon becoming overweight that is an obstruction to losing weight and building a healthy body image. The sense of failure that is sometimes associated with being overweight interferes with goal setting and taking the bold steps to reach the rewarding goals. One must rid oneself of the failure syndrome. Though solutions are initiated in the mind, we see that the self-same resolutions, paradoxically, falter in the mind. No matter. The truth is you can do this if you think you can. Furthermore, you can do this because I know you can. (You may wonder, is this guy super-encouraging, just plain-old positive or totally arrogant? None of that; stay focused.)

As you can program a computer, so can you program your mind. These are very similar mechanisms. This was introduced to us on a practical, everyday level by Dr. Maxwell Maltz in the 1960s in his book, *Psycho-Cybernetics*. He pointed out how we respond to the information we feed ourselves about who we think we are (self-image) and where we are going (goals). If we think of ourselves poorly and set weak or tentative goals, we will stumble about miserably. Conversely, a loving self-image and promising goals reap great rewards.

The wonderful thing is you are in charge. Whatever deep wounds or shrouded misconceptions are responsible for disabling inner thoughts, they need not be painstakingly uncovered. Talking with a psychologist to fix dysfunctions before continuing your weight-loss plans might be wise. However, you yourself can reprogram your mind with healthy images and positive, appropriate goals. Replace old habits of thought with new thinking and resourceful habits. Awareness of the harm of "wrong thinking" and knowing that habits can be reconstructed is the first step.

Practice is the second.

Listed below are areas of thought we entertain regularly with little regard for the emphasis we apply to the negative; just another example of obscure habits eating away at our floorboards like dry rot.

Eliminate the negative and accentuate the positive. You're not fat.

- *I'm not fat; I'm losing weight and building muscle.*

- *I'm not lazy; I'm taking energetic steps toward getting stronger.*

- *I'm not overwhelmed; I'm in the daily creative process of eating right and learning about myself.*

- *I'm not anxious and impatient; I have the rest of my life to get better and better, day by day.*

- *I'm not fearful; I'm strengthening my body, mind and spirit.*

- *I'm not a lost cause; I'm braver and smarter, stronger and more toned today than yesterday.*

- *I'm not on a diet to lose weight; I'm living a joyful, more intelligent and grateful life forever.*

And guess what? Occasionally we make mistakes, which is good because we grow from them every time.

Attitude—how we perceive things—can be learned and un-learned. It takes willful rethinking. Believe it. Take action now.

Look here: *Exercise is boring*. Wrong thinking. It's boring if you think it is. The truth is, exercise is vitally important to your health and well-being. You are accepting a misconception typical of the un-educated masses who, unlike you, will diminish as they continue in their haze. Simple exercise is novel and fun and its qualities of restoration are quickly realized. As you practice and learn the basics with proper guidance and encouragement, a world of growth and promise opens up to you.

The common alternatives to exercise are boring: Sitcoms are boring, tacky, aimless and mind numbing. So are the fattening treats that go with them. Let's not talk about video games that engender anger, violence and anxiety. Exercise is real, exciting and life-giving... with you in control.

*Exercise is hard work.* What's wrong with hard work if you're in control of the output? It's hard work with an appeal that is gratifying to the spirit and rewarding to the body. You are challenged, you overcome; you are fulfilled and you succeed. Everything we need to bloom, to live life in its essence is wrapped up in a workout of 30 to 60 minutes. Training as recommended in these pages builds functional muscle, strengthens the heart and lungs and helps detoxify the system. And do you have any idea how it manages undesirable stress, that sticky black gunk that stores up in your back, neck and personality?

The chain gang doing roadwork in the Mississippi sun... that's hard work. Workouts are a blast.

*Exercise takes too much time.* It does take time: three to six hours a week out of a possible 168. Think. Think of the benefits, my friend. I would list them, but I'd feel silly after number 50. Okay, I'll give you a quick 15: builds muscle, contributes to fat loss, builds strength and shape, strengthens the heart and lungs, diminishes stress, improves endurance, increases energy, increases bone density, adds to sport performance, improves sense of worth and confidence, builds smiles and clears the mind.

Think of the consequences if you don't. I'd list them, but they're depressing. One sorry consequence is the elimination of the short list of benefits above. Don't you think the time is worth it?

I have a friend, 10 years younger than I, who was my training partner 10 years ago. He looked and moved like a professional line-backer. In his mid-30s he grabbed the opportunity to expand his business to include the entire West Coast. "Gonna make some bucks and retire while I'm young and a little crazy." I gave him a lifetime membership and he promised to train with the early morning crowd. The story is not a new one. His business boiled and his workouts evaporated. His finances increased and so did his belly. His back weakened along with his disciplines. The complimentary membership to the gym went unused year after year. He's large today, Type 2 diabetic and occasionally bedridden. It's the gout. He looks old and doesn't get around much anymore. He has lots of time but nowhere to go. "If only I had worked out with the morning crowd," he grunts. I'll drag him to the gym as soon as he's able. Promise. Fix that boy up.

*Weight lifting is for muscleheads.* Yes, yes, yes. Now you're catching on. Musclehead, once considered a slur, is a compliment reserved for the determined and tough, yet ingenuous, men and women who forge onward knowing no other direction or manner of movement. Sometimes this character exists in the least-likely personality and only needs to be jarred loose. With a little luck, there's a musclehead in you.

## The mind is a playground

You have concluded by now that I am not a distinguished professor with an accumulation of degrees from universities. I try to hide the fact, but the word gets out. This does not, however, prevent me from expressing what I think. You ready? A few of you reading this book have extensive physical conditions that inhibit your weight-loss and muscle-building processes. My heart goes out to you as I have my own limiting conditions to provide me with understanding. Many of you who are overweight—substantially, chronically and stubbornly overweight—have problems that originate in your mind and you know it, don't know it or deny it. Whatever the case, they eventually need to be addressed as you seek your healthy shape-up goals.

I would be remiss if I did not underline the value of wise counsel: a pastor, a psychologist or sterling friend. An objective and aware person can reveal subtle, yet baffling, flaws in your mental outlook that thwart your weight-loss progress; and they can support and guide you. Work on both projects, the mind and the body simultaneously, to turn things around.

My foremost therapy is found within my faith, a gift for which I am grateful. Therapy in abundance is found on the gym floor, as well. This may come as a big surprise to you, but I attribute great power to exercise, weight lifting in particular, and rave about its life-enhancing qualities. Oops, let the cat out of the bag that time. The reasons for this are scientific, if anyone gives a hoot, but the proof is in the action. Anyone who spends enough time on the gym floor, or has in the past, knows of what I speak. I believe that no other activity can so dramatically reform and restore you as resistance exercise performed with consistence and diligence.

Listen closely. The secret concoction consists of weight training mixed with a splash of aerobics and just the right amount of good food. Add water and heat and serve generously throughout your lifetime. Do this with a thankful heart.

You'll gain a harmony with yourself if you've never had it or regain it if you've lost it along the way. You'll solve problems, avoid problems and handle problems that once confounded you. You'll kick stones out of your way rather than trip over them. You'll make a friend and take time to help him for his sake rather than your own. You know the fat that has burdened you, shamed you, saddened you and bent you low for so long that you want to scream? You'll acknowledge the fat for the thing it is as you press on at the gym with assurance and might, as you observe its departure from a comfortable distance and get on with your life in all its goodness. Though exercise is physical action, the roots beneath its tenacious trunk grow from the soil of your mind. And the fruit produced from its generous branches serves that same wonderful mind.

Is this dude a farmer, a musclehead or a Looney Tune?

"Okay," you say, "it's in the mind. I'm not into exercise and I'm not going to the gym or run around the block or peddle a silly bike that doesn't move. What do you think of that, Mr. Whatever?"

Got your message. I will continue to persuade, cajole, threaten and humor you in the pages to follow. Stick with me—and the rest of us—as I scratch for solutions and try to make a good situation out of a bad one. Or, you might want to mark the page and place the book on the top shelf. Maybe next year at this time you'll want to pull it down and review it... murmuring with regret, if only....

## University brainstorm

There are highly accredited universities that study the complex issues of obesity and offer clinics to help people overcome their difficulties. One such school of learning has a good success rate because it is legitimate, tries hard and is staffed by credentialed professionals. It also charges an arm and a leg for its elite services... one sure way to precipitate weight loss if all else fails. Here we have the perfect setting for a person, even a doubter, wanting to lose weight. Everything he needs for conviction is stacked before him and he is convinced from the onset it will work. He says to himself secretly, deep in the subconscious where the heavy thinking takes place, "With all this authority and authenticity, and all this heady and professional support, I can not fail to lose weight." The mind at work.

The university experts point out that the difficulty is often in the thoughts and perceptions of the obese. Much of their approach is to untangle mistaken concepts, poor habits, misbehavior and destructive and compulsive tendencies of their clients—things of the mind. Someone in the past has been messing with the customer's personal computer: Mom, "Clean your plate;" Dad, "You can't do that;" Brother, "You're a fathead;" the bully in the third grade pushed you down in front of the girls; the no-neck coach called you "Tubs" and a merciless society calls upon you to look like Superwoman or Joe Polooka.

I cannot and do not disagree. I apply the mind-over-matter technique. Burdened and confused by my own hang-ups, I say take the compulsive tendencies to the gym and *concentrate* on busting them up, beating them down and tearing them apart. I reduce the hang-ups to sets, reps and very effective exercises for building muscle and losing fat. Fortunately or not, most clinics do not advocate DPS, Draper Primal Solutions. Civilized, they tend to nudge, pamper and stroke the pounds away.

## Young mastermind

Jim raises horses on the sunny hillsides of Aptos, a community neighboring Santa Cruz. He's one of the good ole boys, having grown up in New York City and wandering to the West Coast years ago. He's middle-aged and loves his workouts. "They keep me strong, sane and young for an old guy," he says. His daughter, Jesse, helps on the small ranch and is home-schooled. One of her education requirements is physical fitness, which she attains at World Gym. I was concerned about her, not yet a teen and isolated on a farm, learning fence repair, barn hygiene and her ABCs on the back porch. She was shy and a little rough around the edges for a California girl.

She received sufficient encouragement as we put her through the paces of "The Introductory Routine." Her independence glowed like a candle in an otherwise shaded place. Jesse was happy on her own. She remained in my peripheral vision; Jim gave her fatherly teasers to keep her alert and her mom joined her occasionally for the fun of it. She's 15 today, carries herself with natural assurance and speaks thoughtfully and intelligently. Her muscles are supple and strong and they match an optimistic teenage outlook. You get the feeling she won't veer off course because she set it in motion with hard work and lots of undistracted contemplation. She's got a good head on her shoulders.

"You're doing good, girl," I said, displaying my profound guru preciseness and adult masculine charm. "Thanks, Dave. The gym gives me a chance to think about things while I attack the weights. I'm, like, building brains and muscles at the same time. It's real. It's fun. It's cool." I tried to think of something clever to say and gave her a hug instead.

## Crazy, man

I urge you to exercise not because I'm obsessed, can't see past my own fixations and selfishly want you to join me in my madness. Nor am I ignorant of the fact that most people are not exactly crazy about the activity. I simply and strongly believe basic fitness is a personal responsibility, an obligation we should not ignore, a wise investment assuring high dividends and a debt we need to pay to guarantee life-time satisfaction. How many of us like to work from nine to five or hit the cross-town traffic eight in the morning only to turn around and fight our way back at six? It's got to be done or we're on the streets with empty pockets and a tin cup, right? It's no different with exercise and good eating. It's got to be done or we're in the world without strength and health and an engaging attitude.

Physical fitness and good health aren't options; they're necessi-ties. You're not bound by law to be fit, but the personal penalty for its neglect is severe. The gym, exercise and sound eating will mold, re-store, revitalize and preserve you; they accommodate healthy lives and give life to those who abused it.

Training (the term I prefer when speaking collectively of exer-cise, good nutrition and their continual practice) belongs, along with faith, family, friends, cat, dog, home and career, on your Top 10 list. Some people put it after their shiny red Mustang; most people don't put training on their list at all. Incredible, huh?

## Back to the drawing board

I'm about to perform one of my popular magic tricks and bring Dr. Maxwell Maltz back to center stage. I attribute the brilliance (belly laughs acceptable) of my early movements in the '60s to the logic of his principles and have accompanied me since. They are positive think-ing with muscle and might. He introduced me to the *subconscious mind*, which he compared to a servomechanism that responds to your thoughts and imagination. Immediately you respect this silent and invisible partner with its fathomless ability. Don't get nervous at this point as if I were introducing you to the occult or some obscure and weird underground practices. It's just plain old common sense.

Apparently you give your subconscious a job to do and it goes about accomplishing the task, directing you to do small chores to assist in the goal-achieving process. This is done beneath the surface of mental observation, and communication is unconscious and spontaneous. The job the subconscious is required to do is defined by the true image you have of yourself and the real goals you set in your life. Your subconscious makes no judgements; it performs efficiently and impersonally.

Not everyone sits down in the cool of the evening and, while sipping a protein shake, remolds their downcast self-image and lists their hopeful short- and long-term goals. It simply doesn't occur to most folks. They just slug it out day after day knowing they've got a job to do and struggles to overcome. However, should you pursue self-improvement and engage in the process of programming your mind with constructive thoughts, prepare yourself for moving small mountains. It's a creative process requiring imagination and considerable conviction and works better than a beer and Monday night football, or the alternative, tapping your forehead with a ball-peen hammer.

At 21 I migrated from New Jersey to the West Coast. I applied the precepts according to Dr. Maltz as I trained in the early '60s in Santa Monica, California. In those days I read very little of anything, though billboards caught my eye. I didn't talk much and occasionally wondered what to say. Action, I noticed, spoke louder than words. I discovered I had a self-image problem when I left my familiar surroundings in Jersey and was totally on my own in California where communication was popular. The black XXL-hooded sweatshirt I wore during the first month, July, was a dead giveaway.

Can you keep a secret? My early environment and poorly seeded mind sabotaged my self-image and I felt... gasp... inferior. No wonder I weighed 250 pounds at age 20 and could bench press 440. Inferior? I was nullified and mortified. I set about actively and creatively to feed new and appropriate information to my berated, substandard self. I gorged on the weights and spoon-fed my subconscious mind with doses of healthy self-image. It takes time and determined effort—and it works. Just as you witness your body responding to intense workouts, tuna and cottage cheese, so do you see and feel your "self" unfolding from collapse with a regular diet of encouragement and visions of a whole and happy life.

Based on this premise of visualizing, there are two parts to the process of moving ahead in the challenging world outside our own. Construction of a healthy self-image is at the top of the list. On its heels is setting the uplifting goals that appeal to you and that are consistent with the ever-improving picture of who you are.

My short-term goal was significant: to make it through the day. My long-term goal needed work, but it, too, was convincing: to make it through the next day. I eventually extended it to include establishing California residency. I assumed the West Coast profile more each day as my silent and invisible partner—my subconscious—worked diligently in his cranial chambers. Mr. America, Hollywood or career didn't occur to me. The future was anything that hadn't happened already. A sinking rubber duck doesn't plan southerly migrations; I was flapping my wings working on the present.

Doing things was not my weak link. It was thinking that presented a problem. I read and re-read those pages of *Psycho-Cybernetics* that rang a bell, those pages that held revelation or a crystal-clear thought or the essence of something that stirred me. No, it wasn't magic because that doesn't exist, but you're close. I continued to feed my mental experience with detailed, positive imaginings. Visualizing is a natural process, I believe, and we respond to it regularly. Some folks have a greater propensity than others for visualizing. Where imagination is not vivid and consistent, it can be stimulated, that is, practiced effort applied to realistic scenarios with you as the star, lean and capable. If your typical imaginings are not positive, they must be terminated and replaced—reprogrammed.

In other words, don't think of yourself as fat and stupid. You might very well become what you think.

You who are 30 pounds overweight and think you're a beast, you've got some work to do. Don't put off this solid and bold approach. The sooner you reconstruct your thoughts about who you are and where you are going, the sooner the inner workings are activated and neat things start happening. Put that imagination to work while you go about daily life: You're on your way to the gym—visualize a superior workout in detail and the completion of tough and reward-ing sets and reps.

Put aside time before fading off at night and imagine yourself a lighter, leaner and stronger person. Be positive, yet sensible and ma-ture in these visions. Do not imagine burning 50 pounds by next summer and looking like Tarzan… or Jane… as there's no room for a monkey in your jungle. You are far too smart. Imagine yourself eating happily according to plan without deviation or over-consumption. And should you stray in real life, don't belittle or berate yourself and thereby sabotage your invested time and mental rebuilding. Be nice. You're the best friend you've got.

## Obesity and the emotions

The link between obesity and the emotions is tight yet frequently undefined. I've reviewed several books that speak intelligently to the issues of rejection, fear, anger, depression, stress, loneliness and other emotional disturbances and their ties to overeating. The details of each relationship were different, but the themes were similar. The feelings of distress, whether new or chronic, would reach a point where eating was a suitable and temporary relief from their pain; eating and its preparation provided the troubled person with a distraction, a re-ward, gratification, comfort or a sense of being loved.

Food indulgence was a reaction both automatic and habitual. The subjects ate and ate uncontrollably as life confronted them with its daily dose of conflict. Time passed and the weight mounted slowly but surely. The wild thing is that these disorders are common and often invisible to the afflicted overeater.

Recommendations by counselors were made to the over-con-sumers to observe their eating patterns and note those occasions when eating was excessive. Questions were asked. Is it legitimate hunger or do you just plainly and simply eat too much? The exercise often fixed an eat-eat situation by interrupting the activity on the spot or prompted the elimination of the unnecessary eating episodes by the diligent breakdown of a bad habit. Were there abnormal emotions present that triggered the wave of overindulgence?

What transpired in the early impressionable years might in part determine eating behavior today. Recognizing and assessing irregular emotional surges can facilitate their dismantling.

The research was broad and deep, and therapy often disclosed the source of overeating. It did not, however, always fix the problem. Work and discipline were still needed to bring about changes.

We are all a little off-balance in that we are not perfect. And not all that appears to be misbehavior is misbehavior or needs analysis— Nothing work, planning, discipline and healthy pride can't fix.

My approach to the overweight problem, if it stems directly from excessive eating, is to stop it by establishing an orderly and defined eating plan that feeds one healthfully and often so hunger is not a haunting problem. It is backed by sufficient exercise to raise the metabolism as muscles grow, calories burn and fat diminishes. The addition of vigorous activity to a physically dormant schedule improves heart and lung power as it fills the mind with purpose, enthusiasm and clear thinking. The combination of eating and exercise is fundamental, and it consistently corrects a bewildered hormonal system.

Exercise, furthermore, redirects and diminishes stress, fills wasted time with the wisdom of physical investment, burns calories as it replaces cravings and relieves the overwhelming guilt of abuse, neglect and domination by food.

## Discipline rules

About discipline: I don't venture off without it. It's tough, it's austere and I treasure it as if it were a loving family member. That is, I welcome discipline always and I long for it when it's hidden. It resides within and has the dimension and life we give it. Discipline is not mean and self-centered or, rather, no more so than its host.

Rarely do people consider this singular feature without a nagging discomfort as if it was a foreign force that is troublesome, a nuisance between happiness and us, or a punishment in our hunt for freedom and success. This couldn't be further from the truth. Discipline, with its calm energy and enabling might, is the only willing and sane companion to share the daily load. As love is felt in the heart and thought in the head, discipline is carried across the back and shoulders, not as a weight but as a steady, outgoing force. It girdles and protects, drives, pushes and pulls.

What do you think about discipline? People asked that question generally grin and jokingly dismiss it as one of those trick questions asked at parties or as a subjective intangible that's reserved for saints and Olympic champions. We all have it, and with work and healthy pride, we can develop it as we can skill and talent. Your mission is to develop your discipline as you develop your weight-loss habits and to develop your weight-loss habits as you develop your discipline.

Research for *Your Body Revival* has me scanning, examining and underlining diet and exercise-related material from a heap of sources. Where relevant, the authors recognize discipline and call for its practice, yet with swift-footed agility, they dance around the subject. They assume discipline is out of man's field of achievement and go on to suggest small ways he can cheat and still get the job done. Cookies here, chocolates there, fast food less often and in smaller portions and watch those beers. And the exercise programs look like they were fashioned for Barbie doll and her gang. Incidentally, Electro abs don't work, nor do the fat-be-gone creams and pills, rubber sweat girdles or a hypnotic CD collection.

Am I talking to the same audience? Tell me it isn't so. Why would intelligent practitioners, students of the sciences and serious non-fiction writers slide the matter under the rug? Discipline is another classic value we lose when it is no longer encouraged, practiced and, therefore, developed. The powerful internal force is destined to shrivel and die like a seldom-used muscle. A reference to discipline will one day be humiliating and unacceptable; it will join the ranks of politically incorrect notions. This is more than a fight for a slim waistline; it's a fight for an endangered species.

> *Discipline establishes confidence and commands respect.*
> *Discipline is the antithesis of neglect, denial and ignorance.*
> *Discipline is smart, engaging and untiring.*
> *Discipline is loyal and will not abandon its possessor.*
> *Discipline knows no foe.*
> *Discipline is the air beneath the wings, the anchor that secures.*

Fat loss and muscle development are directly proportionate to discipline. It's a cosmic truth.

# Chapter 6

## The Food We Eat:
*Carbs, Protein, Fat, Calories & Calculations*

You can relax for a while. The body is in motion; you're walking and crunching, the heart and lungs are spreading the good word to the rest of the system and you have some big muscle groups undergoing the awesome contractions for which they were designed. The mind is activated, filing and recording and preparing. You're going to recondition this vessel, polish the brass and set the timing. It's going to spin like a top, sound good, feel good and be admired. Time, exercise and good food to fuel a quick and trim body—that's all you need. Let's examine the food factor, shall we?

Where did everybody go? You scattered as if I said the creepy "D" word, diet. What's wrong with the word "diet" anyway? We tend to overreact at the mention of the word like spoiled children, as if we might be denied pleasure, starved, rejected or have our cuddly security blanket taken away. I use the term "diet" often when I refer to one's daily nourishment. It's a good word. You can actually stand on one foot and say "diet" out loud without moving your lips.

All you are going to do is eat more regularly starting with a simple meal in the morning (gotta have breakfast) and a meal every three hours or so until evening. You are going to eat a balance of foods to assure the body of the nutrients it requires and thrives on. You are going to look at society's ignoble downfalls—fast food and junk food—and eliminate them. Here's where the weak roll over and play dead. Just walk around them and move on.

You're going to replace the sugar, excessive carbohydrates and surplus fat in your menu with the delicious and nutritious foods overflowing in the markets today. You're going to eat portions that are sensible and are calculated to lose fat pounds safely and smartly.

You're going to feed your hunger, not your mad cravings or ravenous appetite.

You'll fortify yourself with an attitude that develops self-esteem, strength, energy, endurance and general good looks. You are going to build muscle and might, spirit and enthusiasm.

We are possessed of intelligence, discipline, fortitude and hope. They might register on the low end of the scale right now, but that mark will rise as you turn the pages and grasp each day. Did I mention the key element, desire? If you've got desire, brothers and sisters, you're going a long, long way. It's some kind of mysterious  law of the universe like orbiting planets and gravitational force. Desire rules.

## The language of nutrition

Let's start with some basic words, terms and definitions. By the way, tossing the word obesity around makes me nervous. Here are some standard, overly generalized clarifications:

**Overweight: 10-20% higher than normal weight**
**Obese: 20% or more above normal weight (excess in bodyfat)**
**Morbidly obese: 50-100% above normal weight or 100 pounds**
**over ideal weight**

Now we can get on with the show.

I don't rave about my vast, in-depth knowledge of nutrition, biochemistry and physiology, nor do I apologize for the lack of it. Too much researching and data collecting can obstruct the pursuit and achievement of the noble goals: to lose weight and gain muscle.  But how can we talk intelligently about changing our body weight without including the words metabolism, protein, carbohydrate and fat? Who would understand us without caloric and gram calculations considered? Let's summarize these practical references and look foward to the fine day when we will no longer depend on their preponderance in our minds. Sweet instinct, be our guide.

The famous calorie or, more technically correct, the kilocalorie, is not something you eat. This took me a long time to accept. The calorie is a unit of heat used to calculate the energy in food as well as the energy released in the body. To be precise one calorie is the amount of energy needed to raise the temperature of one gram of water by one degree centigrade. Huh?

The foods we eat are composed of the various nutrients needed to support a healthy and strong body, including protein, carbohydrate and fat. These ingredients, the hugely complex and interdependent macronutrients, provide the vast majority of calories we require for energy, for fuel.

> *Protein ..............1 gram represents 4 calories*
> *Carbohydrate ........1 gram represents 4 calories*
> *Fat .....................1 gram represents 9 calories*

Further, proteins composed of smaller units, or amino acids, intricately build the body. Carbohydrates (carbs) provide most of the fuel for its activity and fats fuel the body and reside within the body's structure to complement its well-being.

Vitamins, minerals (known as micronutrients) and water are vital to life, yet supply no calories. Fiber and cholesterol provide no calories, and one gram of alcohol, a popular non-nutrient found in pouchy beerskies, offer us seven calories.

Metabolism commonly refers to the rate at which the body burns food calories. Everyone has their own rate of metabolism depending on genetics, muscle mass, body weight, activity, system chemistry, age, sex and so forth. The Basal Metabolic Rate, or BMR, is the minimum number of calories required to maintain vital functions (breathing and heart action) while the body is at rest.

• Each of us has a different genetic layout that to some extent decides our calorie-burning, fat-storing and muscle-building characteristics. These are alterable factors, which we can successfully affect by diet and exercise.

• Body composition is a main factor in determining our metabolic rate. Muscle is metabolically active and burns calories whereas fat is inactive and virtually burns none.

• A man generally has 20 percent more muscle than a woman and thus burns up to 10 percent more calories than a woman of the same age, height and weight.

• Regular physical activity increases metabolic rate as calories are burned to support work or sport.

• Metabolism slows down as one gets older. Often this is attributed to decreasing activity and muscle.

• Metabolism slows down when we don't eat.

• A heavier body requires more work (more calories) to maintain and support than a lighter body, resulting in a higher rate of metabolism. This apparent contradiction is explained by the usual presence of more muscle with more weight and more work required in moving more weight; that is, the body presents a greater resistance to the working muscles.

## How many calories do you need?

Sparing the array of convoluted equations for determining adequate daily calories, let's go with a reasonable formula often used by researchers: Body weight in pounds multiplied by 12 to 15 calories. twelve is the number to choose if you're a female with average activity, and 15 is the number for a moderately active male… your call. Remember, these are rough estimations to position us at the starting blocks where the action begins.

If you're a woman weighing 150 pounds and operate a computer in an insurance firm, the math is 150 (pounds) x 12 (calories) = 1,800 calories to keep you going around the clock. An active man of 200 pounds (200 pounds x 15 calories) might require 3,000 calories to get things done. Whoever lifts weights and runs the stairs can add calories according to his or her expert assessment.

To lose body fat, you must burn more calories than you consume. This one, inconspicuous statement is the foundation of almost every weight-loss book on the market. The remaining 50,000 words supplied by the authors only serve as fluff to support it.

One pound of fat contains 3,500 calories. A shortfall of 3,500 calories is needed to lose one pound of fat, theoretically. An appealing plan is to drop 500 calories from your optimum intake each day and expect a deficit of 3,500 calories in seven days or a loss of one pound each week. This is a valid target; that is, you're aiming in the right direction and accuracy will be gained as you practice and account for other variables.

Include adequate aerobic and weight workouts (already underway with the commencement of walks, jogs and midsection exercise, right?) to burn more calories and contribute to your conditioning, and you are manipulating the proper levers and pushing the right buttons to reconstruct your body.

## A quick preview

Throughout my athletic history, I never got into the calorie-counting routine. I have, since the beginning of time, counted grams of protein from meat, fish, poultry, eggs and dairy. One and a half to two grams per pound of body weight has been my target. Carbohydrates come sparingly from al dente vegetables of all varieties, with an accent on the dark in color, and lots of salads. Here we have micronutrients by the truckload. The fruits are held to three pieces a day because of the high simple-sugar content, and I depend on the milk to add to my adequate carb stockpile. Fat is relatively high in my diet as red meat, which affords my favorite concoction of muscle-building aminos, is bountiful, plus I add essential fatty acids (EFAs) to my daily food intake for a variety of healthy reasons that I'll mention later. That's me in a nutshell.

I take a handful of precious vitamins and minerals to compensate for the manhandling and processing of the foods we eat (over-farmed soils, chemically treated livestock and produce, cold-storage denaturing, prematurely picked produce). Protein shakes abound to press more goodness into my system at key times throughout the day; I lug a jug of water wherever I go.

I can calculate the grams of each nutrient and come up with totals at the end of the day. 4,000-5,000 calories, depending—they vary with my activity and, truthfully, I seldom do the math. The interesting thing is my ratio: 40-percent protein, 30-percent carbohydrate and 30-percent fat. I like that. The standard material from today's nutritional counselors and dietitians tells me to eat more grains and about 25 percent of my total calories from protein. I don't think so. Okay for elevator operators but not for us aiming to be lean. Protein rules.

## Insisting on listing

Do you automatically have a pad and pencil ready? You'll need to make some references. I highly recommend you record all the foods you eat and their values through the days ahead. Lists compiled at the day's end or on the spot take on a life of their own and when you jot down things that are ugly and unexplainable (chocolates, fries, six-pack), they glare at you. I am not fond of things that glare at me. Serious weight-loss practitioners, powerlifters and bodybuilders prove that lists, notes and records work. It'll take patience to follow your daily patterns and calculate nutrient portions, grams, calories and percentages. It's a good practice early on. As you become familiar with common values, develop honor and trust the process, you can relax the reins. Today, the pad and pencil are weight-loss tools as effective as barbells, dumbbells and sneakers.

Confidentially, I grow weary when it comes to being too exact with the calculations. This is where some folks go AWOL, skip bail, jump ship, crash and burn or otherwise quit. The nagging sense of limitation, measured freedom and burdensome factoring drive a wedge between the living person and the living goal. I do believe a clear understanding of the facts and figures put forth will serve you extremely well—discipline worn on your sleeve. However, detailed computations can become preoccupying and you might lose focus of the good task at hand. Be careful. They are important but not to be worshipped. They are gauges; let them guide you, and do not mistake them for the exercise itself.

Ultimately, fat loss is not in the details and minutia; it's in the solid and bold work.

I love order. Reviewing the fundamentals organizes the mind and arranges related thoughts in a neat row. Summarizing supports credence and confidence, ingredients seldom held in excess. Revision is challenging and engaging and calls upon courage. During the early phases of planning and applying, you are nurturing commitment, as well. The old foundation, cracked and neglected, needs restoring if the new structure is to stand. You are entering the hard-hat area. Watch your step. Mind the gap.

# Chapter 7

## Food Factoring:
### *Keeping Track of Yourself & the Food You Eat*

I see some restless bodies pulling at their collars, yawning, staring at the clock and muttering, "Let's get on with it, already."

Good. We agree that you need to make some references and I highly recommend you record all the foods you eat and their values through the days ahead. Bite the bullet. I suggest you pick up a convenient calorie counter at your local bookstore and keep it handy. Here's another popular approach: "Be still. Starting now you're keeping records or else."

Over a total of four days, including one weekend day, eat as you please in order to prepare a record of your typical eating habits and approximate food intake. List the foods and their portion size and make notes of any stimulating thoughts and feelings that might assist you in the operation. Again, the recordings can be done on the spot or at the day's end—your choice—as long as accuracy is sure. Translate foods into grams of protein, carbohydrate and fat and, finally, calories. When the four-day project is complete, total the calories and the grams of the individual nutrients. Divide by four and you'll have your average daily consumption.

I'm with you. Right about now I twitch and my mind wanders. I start pacing and say with tight lips, "Where's the iron?" I hope you're with me and anxious to roll, but these calculations are essential. We can no longer go on guessing, pretending or blundering. What we eat, how much and when, largely determine our obesity and health.

Exercise works hard to form our mass into a shapely, strong and vigorous body. The two work together like rock and roll, rhythm and blues, jazz and cool; it's music, man.

You still walking, slow running and working your midsection like you promised? I want you in shape. You're about to perform the calorie-juggling trick and the food-balancing act. You are about to confront the naked truth.

I present you with 11 ideas to toss around as the grams, calories and percentages unfold and you develop a profile:

**1.** Begin by arranging an eating schedule starting with breakfast as meal one and eating every three hours throughout the day until bedtime. In fact, I'll provide a day's menu with recommended foods and their nutrient breakdown, grams, calories and proportions. You'll get the hang of it if this business of dropping fat and building muscle really matters. It's work, demands commitment, challenges discipline and requires compromise. Those who lurk in the shadows will think you're crazy, but you're on a mission.

**2.** What in your menu looks nasty, dumb or scary? Seriously consider its elimination. Start by clearing the refrigerator, kitchen cabinets and counter tops of the obvious undesirables: pop, potato chips, cookies, worthless sugary cereals, white bread, crackers and Ding Dongs. The donuts go; hotdogs, frightening sausages, chocolate cream puffs, candy corn from Halloween and the Pop-tarts on the bottom shelf... they're out. Give them to the neighbor's mangy dog, the one that barks all night... that'll keep him busy.

Remove the source of calories, temptation, guilt, failure and disappointment and stuff it in a large, plastic garbage bag. Out of sight, out of mind. You'll be amazed how housecleaning refreshes your purpose and contributes to your cause, to say nothing of tidying the funky kitchen.

**3.** Take pleasure and pride in replacing the empty space created by the clean sweep with tuna, cottage cheese, yogurt, nonfat milk, fresh wholesome vegetables, fruit in abundance and variety, poultry, lean cuts of meat and eggs. Learn to read labels and shop wisely. Never shop for food when you're hungry and not without a prepared list in hand. Do not flirt with seductive, syrupy, gooey foods, lest you be tempted. That stuff will surely lead you down the road to ruin.

**4.** Do you think you could trim down the serving size on this one, Judy? I suggested a piece of fruit for meal three. My goodness, girl, that's a watermelon you've got your arms wrapped around and a Costco-size tub of cottage cheese on your lap.

Smaller portions will satisfy your energy and muscle-building needs. It doesn't matter what you're eating, even too much protein at one sitting overworks the system and stores fat. Gluttony leads to destruction.

**5.** The question all along the way as you walk and jog toward your streamlined image is how hard are you willing to work? How much will you extend yourself, apply discipline and sacrifice before you fold? Depends on who you are, how serious you are and how strong you are. Also, it depends on how you define discipline and sacrifice. Seems to me if work is approached with desire, purpose and the right attitude, sacrifice takes on a luster and sparkle of its own. Sacrifices are gemstones, not burdensome, low-grade ore. Living with discipline is a joy in itself. Willpower, once developed, is like an extra pair of hands, a willing servant and a cheerful holiday; it frees you to run and jump or just sit still in peace.

**6.** Eating out can be an adventure, a treat, a memorable occasion or a wonderful experience. I believe it's one of our favorite pastimes, an intimate time where soft emotions are stimulated and sharing begins. Unless, of course, you're at a fast-food joint where the race is on and stuff resembling food is tossed around as if you were in a blaring TV game show. The objective: how much you can eat in the shortest period of time. The prizes: ketchup, mustard and mayonaise in the hair and a rolly polly belly.

You are always able to eat relatively well, if not extraordinarily well, at almost any restaurant. Going through the menu making smart choices is no longer uncommon in the diet-conscious culinary landscape. There's always lean meat, vegetables and salad. If a hitch exists, it's usually in the patron whose appetite is brimming over and self-control is at home in the closet.

Remember, before you go to bed, list all foods ingested—in detail, down to the last crouton.

**7.** Drink water. Pure water is worth more than pure gold. Savor it and drink it by the jugs all day long. If you're not so sure about your tap water, invest in your favorite water bottling company or in a Brita water filter.

**8.** There's no shortage of delicious protein sources on our menu, therefore a protein supplement is optional. However, the efficiency of frequent eating and the demand for a high-protein intake to build muscle persuade me to include a good protein powder for convenience and timing. It is quick food and very nutritious if blended with milk or juice, fresh fruit and some ice; a great breakfast, pre-workout and post-workout meal or a simple shake-in-a-jar if you're on the road. As you watch the calories and when activity is low, mix it with water only.

Meal replacement bars are okay in a pinch, but don't expect them to substitute for a meal. Add it to tonight's calorie list. I'm not the slightest bit crazy about the popular, broadly advertised, pre-mixed meal replacements in a can. That's a "no."

**9.** The *Standard Balanced Menu* discussed later will provide you with a wide assortment of vitamins and minerals that work hard to keep you alive and well. In addition, to ensure total coverage, I advocate a top-quality vitamin and mineral formula that is balanced, carefully processed under low temperature and microencapsulated for timed release.

**10.** You're making progress as you read, but the concrete steps commence when you put the book aside and apply the principles. The truth is in the application, and application doesn't cease unless your vision and desire cease. An absurd thought, isn't it?

Here is a spatter of related questions to stir your appetite… er… rather, stir your thinking: When will you work out, how often and for how long? Where will you train and what will you do? Do you believe in exercise? Will you exercise alone or with a friend? I'll make suggestions and prod you along the way, and there are outlines and exercise descriptions in the chapters ahead.

I'll encourage you to be creative, experiment and improvise because you are capable and because necessity demands it. The pump is near.

**11.** About cheating: You are a responsible individual and anything you do that resembles cheating in diet, exercise or behavior is a temporary malfunction. Your goals are in place and it's your goals that lead you. You're not seeking perfection and you know very well that mistakes, though masterful instructors, make lousy bedfellows. We forever weed the garden and attend the blossoms. Keeps us humble and content.

## Say "Hi" to Reg

I have a friend, call him Reg, who three years ago at 5'10" and age 41, weighed 330 pounds. Dieting wasn't new to him, as he had lost 150 pounds twice at different phases of his life on a mix of radical fad diets (Atkins, liquid, low protein-low calorie and walking, fasting), only to gain the weight back when he blinked. While supporting twice the body weight than one should, there are numerous problems one suffers, from general inertia and system overload to diabetic symptoms and physical and emotional disability. At 330 it's just plain tough to get out of bed in the morning.

One cold winter Reg saw his weight reach an all-time high and he imagined he had chest pains. The big guy sat down—once again—to consider his growing predicament. A year into 40, the occasion was more solemn than ever before.

"Diet? Which one this time?

Fasted through the summer, lost 30 pounds and got weak as a baby. That's out.

How long has it been since my last try? A month? Six weeks?

The high-carb diet was my winter plan and I gained over 20 pounds. Not going there again.

The Atkins diet worked, but no carbs is too strict. Don't know about all that fat.

What did I weigh when I started and how much did I lose?

Sixty pounds in six months, down to 250, I think... or was that the year before?

Reg was troubled. A chill of desperation, something new to the man, dashed through his overgrown body. "Gotta make a move, can't go on like this; nothing makes sense. Where do I begin? What do I do?"

He noticed for the first time he was reviewing and questioning his track record, and an impressive set of footprints had he made. Nearly resigned to extraordinary largeness, "My fate," Reg pulled out a pad and pen to note his observations more definitively.

A list formed. He never lacked discipline or fortitude. His success at losing hundreds of pounds during his yo-yo-dieting career was proof of that. He diligently implemented a dozen different diets;  he had experience and practice.  Interestingly, some worked, some were appealing and some almost killed him. But, what was their structure, the reasoning behind them? The notations grew.

He'd never seen a diet outline or details intelligently laid out. His previous weight-control attempts were based on random input that filed into his mind from some vague floating sources: Reader's Digest, May 1986, a dog-eared "liquid-diets-that-work" book (passed on by a friend), an inspiration from Becky one morning at the office coffee machine. Great. He never had a plan and nothing was ever charted. His nutritional landscape was a vast, barren wasteland. Here he had something tangible, almost tenable: curious notes based on a haze of experience and evaluations, his own. He needed more. His sedentary computer lifestyle was his downfall, but it served to provide easy access to Internet research and knowledgeable websites that made clear to him that resistance exercise, particularly lifting weights, was a big missing variable in his equation.

The order, the clarity of penciled thought, the lingering at the pad for long moments of hopeful musing, the reassurance of his own still presence and the steely sense of the next step to take convinced him: "This is going to work. Weights for muscle, high protein for the muscle building, the right carbs at the right time; fats are okay. I'll take some measurements, track my progress, list my daily food intake and make notes regularly. Find the body weight that I can appreciate that allows me to be strong, look good and continue building muscle, muscle, muscle. I don't need the perfect weight; I just need to do this. Stand back, everybody, I'm loose."

Reg observed that the junk food and fast food were the most frightening presence in his heavy life. He always ate plenty of good food, but the bad food reached shameful proportions. These went first. He rearranged his eating to allow three hours between meals of high protein, medium carbs and medium fat. This practice alone eliminated hunger and craving from his life. Minus the junk the big guy had dropped 2,000 sloppy calories and buckets of chemicals, sugar and salt. He ceased retaining lakes of water and his hormones behaved more agreeably. His heart, now less burdened, supplied endless energy and the pending threat of diabetes abated. Fat storage became less of a problem and muscle synthesis took hold on a regular basis.

Today, calculations estimate a comfortable 40-30-30 balance (40 percent of Reg's calories are derived from protein, 30 percent from carbohydrates and 30 percent from fat). At 210 pounds, Reg is very happy, zigzagging between 3,500 and 4,000 calories to match a high-intensity, zigzag lifting program, his favorite technique of the day. "I'm in the best shape of my life and I love my lifting. The weights are going up and I feel good." His head is on his shoulders as he sits before his computer solving other people's problems and resting from his early morning workout. His son wants to be just like his dad when he grows up.

You still there? Hello... wake up. We're having a quiz. How hard will it be to drop the unnecessary calories, schedule your meals, increase the protein, calculate a reasonable macronutrient balance and stick to the plan? Will you do it? Grade yourself. Thank you. You're dismissed.

# About Water

*Old miner's mule song*

*Water me down in the mornin',*
*Slosh my buckets middle of the day,*
*Wet my thirsting body toward evenin'*
*Lest my bones go dry and I blow away.*

We are roughly two-thirds water, depending on muscle mass, gender and age. And, no, we don't drink enough to satisfy our needs. We lose water all day through the skin, breath and elimination of waste. Half of us are mildly hypo-hydrated and, therefore, we compromise the body's functions—and our performance. We push the body like thoughtless masters, yet we survive because the body is incredible.

Water provides vital service to every cell, moving food from the first bite, through the digestive process, into the blood and into the cells as nutrients, and, finally, out as waste.

Water is crucial to maintaining body temperature, lubricating joints and giving fullness and shape to cells. Deny the system adequate water and we exhibit symptoms of dehydration, including fatigue, headache, dry throat and stiffness. There's hopeful research that says water by the quarts might dilute the risks of certain cancers, including breast, colon and bladder cancers. I'm reminded as I write to grab my handy water bottle and take a long sweet drink. Join me?

We lose at least two quarts of water a day, much more if it's very hot or we are very active.

Replenishment comes via the watery foods we eat and the liquids we drink. Larger people obviously need more water proportionately to accommodate the larger metabolic loads.

While few people ingest enough of the clear liquid, most folks insist on mixing it with sugar, flavorings, chemicals and caffeine. The chemicals we surely don't need and which may be toxic, the sugar spikes our insulin and is a generous source of unwanted calories, and the caffeine has diuretic properties that negate the drink's hydrating effects.

Eliminating soft drinks and their counter-point companion, salty chips, from the diet is a giant step toward good health and fat reduction. Sugar spikes insulin and disturbs a string of hormonal responses that support fat storage. Salt promotes unnatural, extra-cellular water retention—bloat.

Here's your chance to make a small, yet significant commitment and take a giant step toward your goals—health, fat loss and discipline: Drink more water.

Avoid calorie-dense juices as thirst quenchers and hydrators. Though they contain some nutrients, the sugar content might be too high a price to pay. Often, commercially processed juices are profanely altered and the goodness has been replaced by something weird.

Often we think we're hungry, but we're actually thirsty. If you drink only when you're thirsty, you're late; thirst comes upon us when we're already half a quart low on fluids. Drink regularly throughout the day and consume two quarts of the miracle agent to be safe. You'll get a Gold Star for trying.

*Continued...*

Pretend some kind and wealthy admirer is depositing $10 into your life savings for every quart you drink, redeemable only in old age. The returns will be plentiful; you'll be rich beyond your imagination.

You'll want to know that a plentiful water supply:

- blunts the appetite,

- facilitates fat burning,

- promotes muscle building,

- fights muscle loss,

- readily encourages shift of energy source from glycogen to fat,

- cleanses the cellular system of toxins and waste,

- prevents water retention.

A sufficient water presence in the system promotes the fat-burning process by flushing out the natural fat-burning byproducts via the kidneys.

Further, the kidneys cannot function efficiently without enough water and thus transfer certain aspects of the workload to the liver. The liver's primary job, metabolizing stored fat into usable energy, is hampered and fat storage increases, fat use for energy decreases and glycogen for energy increases (interfering with our low-carbohydrate scheme to fuel the body).

The high-protein diet that is emphasized in these pages is dependent upon water for its cleansing of urea, a waste product of protein metabolism. The greater the ingestion of protein, the more urea leaving the body as urine.

Research shows that as cells increase in volume in response to adequate hydration, an anabolic (muscle building) environment is created. Conversely, as cells shrink due to decreased hydration, a catabolic (muscle breakdown) response is stimulated. Cortisol levels increase with dehydration, a cell-damaging condition.

Water retention is often the symptom of a struggling system. One's first guess would be there is too much fluid entering the body. Logical, but wrong. The more water you drink, the less you retain. In contrast, the less you drink, the more you retain. The vessel in which you dwell insists on surviving and recognizes low levels of water intake as a threat to its life. Any precious incoming water is held selfishly in supply outside the cell walls for its future subsistence and appears as swollen tissue due to the water retention. Drinking more water is the solution to the hoarding.

Confused? Drink at least two quarts of delicious, water a day and turn up the music. Carry it wherever you go. Makes a good habit and serves as a physical reminder of who you are and of your mission. Cheers!

# Chapter 8

## Yo-yos & Fad Diets:
### *Hurt, Damage & Destroy*

I'm not addressing an ordinary bunch of extra-large people who just rode in on the all-you-can-eat cabbage truck. You've contemplated your overweight condition for a long time and have mechanically attached yourself to a fad diet or two. Alluring fad diets and quick fixes flash across the covers of sexy magazines sitting conspicuously at the checkout counters of our colorful and prosperous supermarkets. Billions of dollars are spent annually to beat the overweight rap and, meanwhile, the solution is free, simple and never changes. You know the answer, right? Hint: Exercise and eat right for good.

There are numerous overweight conditions in which the sufferer's health and function have been extremely compromised and active solutions are difficult and complicated. Still, with modified approaches everyone can edge forward to gain a foothold on the slippery slope.

I expect, too, that many of you who are reading *Your Body Revival* have put in your time and are in very good shape hoping only to sharpen your edge. Having trained regularly for years, you are now negotiating the loss of the last persistent pounds. I understand. Progress seems to slow down to a halt as you get in better and better condition. You don't know whether to smile or scream.

The trendy menu, the new-wave approach and the latest Hollywood diet sensation offer low-cal eating plans somehow reworded to pinch you in the bottom and get you moving again. Absolutely every diet in which you eat fewer calories than you burn will work. It's simple physics. And every diet that promises you the body of the robust model will be more or less applied. It's simple psychology. Beware. These have the life span of a mosquito. The schemes last for three days—four at the most—until physical and emotional gravity pull you down. You yawn and fidget and grumble and fold, again.

The crash plans may not be healthy, but you will lose weight. The pounds will come off, but you'll lose muscle and vitality. Trendy fad diets do not work long term because they underfeed the dieter and exercise is not exactly included in the package. He or she loses muscle along with fat and the valuable fat-burning metabolic qualities which muscle provides. Strength, energy and endurance evaporate due to low fuel, lost muscle, insufficient protein and micronutrient ingestion. Resistance fades with the immune system and infection hovers like a vulture. The body, hoping to survive the trauma of starvation, begins to hold fat—a calorie-pinching miser.

Women are considerably more susceptible to fad diets and the yo-yo syndrome than men; hence, the choice of my demonstration model. The perky "Miss Glamour" diet plays havoc with blood sugar and hormones and the hopeful dieter is soon irritable, moody and ailing with low-grade malaise. In time toxins leech into the bloodstream and her face breaks out and her body aches. Calcium leaves the bones. The deterioration is shocking. The body, with its marvelous mechanics and miraculous will to survive, does survive, but the cost is punishing.

She resists forfeiting her weight-loss endeavor, yet resumes eating when the diet takes its toll. She eats and revives; she eats and regains the lost weight. She weighs about the same as when she started the smiley diet some months ago, only she has lost muscle due to dreadful nutrition, and gained stubborn fat as her body responded to signs of starvation. The defeat, the failure and the disappointment add significantly to the stress, and the overweight condition becomes a wound. But they *promised*. Misplaced trust, confusion and emotional turmoil are bullies and play no minor role in her life.

The next weight-control attempt is as devastating, and she is skeptical, hesitant and lacks commitment. She has a new toy. It's the yo-yo.

The yo-yo is not fun. She finds herself at random intervals proceeding down a tenuous path that goes nowhere, really, up and down and around. It's tormenting, frustrating and demoralizing. Inadequate, poorly planned weight-loss programs defeat her as she loses surface weight only to gain it back along with some company. We all know people who have diminished because they failed over and over again. Their self-esteem, with their expectations and dreams, deteriorated. Paradoxically, food often becomes their eventual shelter and shield, a real imprisonment.

Why don't they work... any of them... ever? Fad diets don't work long term because of the following reasons, which I will invent as we go along:

• The dieter is a hopeful and trusting individual who is quick to throw his innocence off the nutritional cliff. Disappointment beats him up and he breaks into a hundred pieces when he lands on the rocks below. Some weight loss was achieved and retained for almost 48 hours before the dehydrated and half-starved body and the emotionally derailed personality fights its way back to its familiar and comfortable ground. Nobody prepared the ambitious dieter for the temporary nature of the charming weight loss. He experiences defeat and is cut deep.

• The groping individual is heavily invested in the overweight condition and a quick-fix fad diet is not sufficient in style or approach for serious weight loss. The recommendations from the popular monthly publication (featuring an attractive couple running down the beach) are appealing and mild, but for this reader metabolic changes are necessary and more advanced strategies need to be designed and implemented. Bigger strategies for bigger bodies.

• The menu offered is food to serve the fledgling dieter who is tiptoeing through the day with a minimum of activity. The calories have been reduced to a number just above basal metabolic requirements (the number of calories to provide enough energy to breathe and keep the heart beating) and suggest nothing of exercise beyond minor everyday activity. Nothing in the way of muscle building is encouraged.

• The more aggressive diets that include exercise suggest the classic aerobics that improve the cardio-respiratory system, heighten the metabolism and add luster to the participant. A few pounds are lost and we have discovered a nice maintenance routine. I shrug and say, " Fine." Aerobics alone do little to build muscle, and too much cardio interferes with healthy muscle development. The real fat hangs on and muscle mass again is neglected.

• Diets suggesting too few calories can cause low blood sugar and the symptoms that accompany hypoglycemia: sluggishness, drowsiness, irritability, jitters and the more serious condition of fainting. The body operating on excessively low calories runs the risk of shifting into a starvation mode where calories are hoarded to preserve the system and are stored as fat. Not what the dieter had in mind.

• The diets that are applauded and revered by the heart, cancer and diabetic associations are very nicely balanced but somewhat upside down for anyone who would like to do a little more than walk about and do their daily thing. We need to be more physical and we need more protein and less sugar to accommodate the muscle-demanding activity of an inspired life.

Brief rant... The profile of society changes as knowledge and understanding grow. It also shifts with politics, the economy and the subtle, apparently innocuous invasion of devious thinking (hype advertising, media spin, lobbyist interests in Washington). Pause and look around, a precious freedom we sometimes fail to exercise. Too often I fall in line and believe everything I'm told.

Point in fact: There are some archaic notions disguised as fact, especially in the area of nutrition. I am not alone in my belief that the various governmental regulations and guidelines concerning nutritional standards are plain wrong. Today's serious, enlightened researchers are frowning on sugar, embracing protein and admit that fat is not the slippery monster it has long been portrayed to be. For over 50 years the government agencies that keep us informed have offered us outdated information that compromises our health. Keep your eyes open. The world is changing.

• "Diet" suggests a relatively short-term menu plan adopted to establish or re-establish a healthy weight from which we can resume our misguided eating habits. The assumption is that fixing the number of pounds we read on the scale also fixes the body and its distressed system that has submitted to overeating the wrong foods over an extended period of time. Sound eating is forever.

The word "diet" originally comes from the Greek word "diaita," which means "manner of living." Balancing protein, carbohydrates and fats, along with the quality of the foods we eat, comprise only a part of the whole. Much more needs to be added to the "manner of living" to make the picture complete—activity and attitude, for example. Restoring and maintaining the health of the system is a gradual, long-term process that requires time, a lifetime of time.

• Fad diets match the slow-to-commit and capricious nature of mankind today. We shuffle along. We dabble and wait for the latest promise. Something faster and easier is surely right around the corner, honest… and at half the price.

Do you realize that the qualities you admire—healthy body weight, strength, muscle and fitness—are attainable? Yes, they are. Do you realize that you cannot attain them without hard work and perseverance? No, you can't. Hard work and perseverance define accomplishment. No good thing is accomplished without them. Could I bestow you with gifts, you would need no others than hard work and perseverance. They are the crown jewels.

## Fad diets

Over the last 30 to 40 years, as the fast-food industry and high-tech phenomenon crystallized and as the fitness industry and overweight phenomenon coincided, diet material of every description has appeared in bookstores and magazine stands everywhere. Some have been million-sellers and others disappeared only to reappear a month later under a different title by another author. Have I joined the ranks? It would appear that way, but I'd rather be set adrift in outer space or swallowed whole by an anaconda than add to the diet show with another song and dance.

Some of the popular writing is superfluous and only skin deep.

However, many of the books on diet by the major publishers are crammed with valuable information and a large number of self-published offerings are brilliant and enlightening.

Is something wrong? The questions evidently have not been answered; the problem obviously has not been solved. Is something missing?

Conjecture... Could it be the author's lack of conviction and inspiration in conveying the vital importance of the nutritional regimens and the consequences one faces when they are not applied? The authors are primarily educators with information to present and they hope that, given the facts, the reader will assimilate them, put them into effect and enjoy the results.

Or, could it be the unwillingness of the reader to listen and apply the recommendations with any seriousness for any significant length of time, in fact, with occasional modifications, a lifetime? Despite the author's passion, it is not the author's function to see that the job gets done. The job is up to you.

Finally, in each book exercise gets a pat on the back, a pinch on the cheek and is escorted to the bench. We'll get to you some other time, Jocko. Kiddos, men and women, if you are sincere, earnest and not given to weakness of character, you will exercise. Regular, consistent, weight-resistance exercise is not optional. It is not conjecture. The train thing is the main thing.

### *Extra. Extra. Read all about it. Muscles rule.*

Weight training is for the macho dudes in tank tops and their airhead girlfriends in tights, something you out-grow by 30. Wrong. Weight-resistance exercise is the smartest, most direct way to fully work the muscles of your body in the least amount of time.

Wherever I have the opportunity, though it might compromise the literary continuity of the book, I will re-mind you of the message, not just the facts, but also the truths.

Think muscle—I'm referring to those muscles that you no longer use and that are diminishing because of the lifestyle you've assumed—the same muscles that allow you to perform daily tasks with ease, the muscles that account for your youthful shape and tone. Muscle is directly re-sponsible for the body's improved resistance to injury and increased ability to absorb oxygen. Muscle and its proper-ties remove limits from your potential and add years to your life. Muscle is vital and, unlike fat, demands energy as it serves its many functions; muscle burns calories.

Ladies, might I remind you that building oversized muscle is not a realistic possibility for you? Fear not. Trim, lovely, strong and shapely, yes. Huge, no. Muscle is dense and will only be displayed as shape and tone. Any increase in bulky size is from an increase in body fat from excessive calorie intake or unbalanced eating that might disturb the hormonal system. Since I'm throwing out the reminders, aerobics do not build muscle. Excessive aerobics can in-terfere with its growth.

Sports in which one participates after the early school years are usually seasonal and infrequent. Studies show that they are responsible more for injuries and accidents than healthy conditioning. They don't come close to accom-plishing the robust and long-lasting effects of gym workouts.

I must have communicated in these pages somewhere how much fun and how fulfilling the gym can be once you get past the typical "cold-steel" impression. No? Sit down, pull up a chair and make yourself comfortable. Can I get you a glass of water? It's like this... when I was kid no bigger than a... blah, blah...

## Diets: The good, the bad and the ugly

Let's take a brief look at the popular mainstream diets:

•Most of the dieting recommendations from the rank-and-file dieticians and nutritionists are consistent with the guidelines of the United States Department of Agriculture (USDA) and the Department of Health Management and Resources(HMR): big on the carbs, low on the fat and light on the protein. They push the grains like they worked in the fields. They distrust fat as if there were only the saturated fats that clog arteries, and protein is given honorable mention for its vague handiwork in the body. It is a meek approach to eating and not designed for the physically aggressive. It is, of course, far better than the diet of the masses of the modern, industrialized nations, but only because their daily food intake is so large, so unbalanced and so loaded with ugly fat, sugars and chemicals—so disastrous.

•The diets that count on food-combining techniques to support their fat-loss claims are not based on fact, only on ill-conceived logic. They claim that certain enzymes are required to healthfully digest certain foods and they will interfere with one another causing digestive disorders or worse if organized food combining is not addressed. Not. It's a fact that enzymes work independent of one another when digesting various foods and do not interrupt the digestive process as a whole. The diets might appear to work well enough, but only based on their relatively low-calorie composition and the early stage eagerness of the dieter.

•Atkins is not far from the target, though too restricted. While the fat freedom is healthy, novel and fun, ingesting protein exclusive of any carbohydrates is really difficult to grasp. The way before the dieter becomes a tightrope across Niagara. Throw in ketosis and the ketone sticks and most folks pack up and go home.

•Cabbage soup has its merits as a raw leap from the catastrophe of fast foods to a featureless menu and mighty-stiff discipline. An overweight, overfed man or woman can endure this abrupt, attention-getting program for a few days to clean the slate and ready him or her for a sensible diet. No doubt a little system cleaning, as well, is a beneficial extra. Sort of a fast without the fast. In two or three days you can bring on the high-protein whole foods in equally spaced meals and reasonable portions. You feel fresh and clean internally and psychologically. A good head start.

•I'm not dead-set against certain short-term, single-food diets (tuna and water, anyone?) that are suddenly installed in a healthy, overstuffed and aware dieter's menu: to shock the system, stir up the hormones and make a statement about earnest commitment. The system is overloaded, well-stocked with nutrients and needs a break. As long as marathons aren't in the immediate schedule, they make a decent introduction to the menu plan I suggest in the following chapter.

•Short-term fasting has enough proponents to save it from the wastepaper basket. Its virtues lie in discipline and the detoxifying qualities. Problems might arise if the poisons in the system channel in the bloodstream causing illness. Muscle breakdown is a sure risk. Be aware; there are smarter ways to go.

•Mini-diets offering flat tummies and tight buns with young starlets demonstrating the bend-at-the-waist exercises are sure yo-yo makers. These are the toys of weight-loss anonymous. Housewives and girlfriends pass these cute darlings around like morsels of gossip. Mini-diets contribute considerably to the casual attitude people have toward fat accumulation. Fads become commonplace, conventional and convenient. There's hope-hype and the quick-fix on every other page. Tomorrow is the day to start the coolest, surest, trendy diet. The pages are brightly pictured with a lovely mom or a gorgeous young model in perfect attire, makeup, lighting and background. She eats grapefruit and yogurt and drinks green tea. The menus are extremely low calorie, and the disciple staggers near starvation. The diets don't last long: lifespan 24 to 48 hours before it's time for a small binge. The magazine to the left suggests cottage cheese and all the fruit you can eat: lifespan four days and the participant gains three pounds. She doesn't diet again for a month or more. They don't work. They discourage. They are pervasive. Yo-yos are forever.

•I applaud *The Metabolic Diet* by Mauro Di Pasquale and the *Natural Hormonal Enhancement* procedures by Rob Faigin. I explain in brief their nutritional position later on in *Your Body Revival.* It's protein all the way, fats are good and excessive carbs are problematic.

• The Zone is a good working diet, light years ahead of the popular, wacky, fad programs running loose in the streets.

As I speak into the bullhorn at worldwide fat-loss rallies, you can clearly hear me call out, "Bring up the protein, ladies and gentlemen, and move the exercise into the foreground. Drop the sugars a little… a little bit more… down, down… there ya go. Just right. Get some rest. See ya at the gym in the morning, ladies and gentlemen. We're rolling."

# Chapter 9

## Boring Menus:
### *Standard Balanced Menu*

What's a book on weight loss without a chapter of boring menus and low-calorie dessert recommendations? Let's start with a plate of carrot sticks, celery stalks and cut clusters of broccoli and cauliflower. Yum, and original, too.

Better yet, in the following pages I outline my exact daily menu to nourish my 6-foot, 225-pound, 59-year-old frame (circa 2002). Incidentally, I train four days a week using weight resistance exercise for 90 to 120 minutes a session.

I've read a number of popular, mainstream, weight-control books recently. Cartoons, charts, graphs and considerable information are presented for the reader to establish a sensible program to lose unhealthy weight. The writers are registered dieticians with noteworthy endorsements and no small staff to support them. I wondered as I read what they were like, what they ate and what they did for exercise. I was curious whom it was who spoke to me about so significant a subject. Of what vine in their life had they picked to provide the sweet ripe fruit of thought? Had they tilled the land and done the planting on their own? Had they nurtured the soil, pruned the branches and seen the seasons come and go as crops failed, were blighted or flourished? Perhaps you are as curious about me.

### Some things never change

The following bill of fare has an uncanny resemblance to my

eating plan of 30 years ago. My menu is another powerful tool in my achieving and maintaining a strong, healthy and enduring body.

Close approximations of nutrient quantities and values have been listed for you to compare to your own records, vague or precise as they may be. I repeat: It is a smart part of your weight-loss plan early on to record your food intake and understand food values and portion sizes. The practice will teach you the basics as you guess serving sizes and fumble with your calorie-counting reference. It is another refining discipline and solid effort, another worthwhile compromise, one more slowing down to note and reinforce your noble goals. I don't doubt many of you already have the techniques polished and apply them automatically.

Ready? Are you wearing your bib? Try not to spill your milk or get crumbs all over the place. This is my daily menu; I plan approximately three hours between meals.

## Draper's Standard Balanced Menu

### Breakfast (meal one):
*Protein shake (comprised of 20 oz. low-fat milk, 1 small banana, 2 large raw eggs, 4 scoops whey-casein protein powder and ice, blended)*
*1 cup coffee with half-and-half*
*1 medium bran muffin, or slice of whole-wheat toast, or cup of oatmeal or granola*

### Mid-morning (meal two):
*10 oz. low-fat milk*
*6 oz. tuna from can*
*1 medium red bell pepper*
*1 slice whole-wheat bread*

### Lunch (meal three):
*10 oz. low-fat milk*
*6 oz. grilled lean hamburger*
*1 medium red potato (microwaved)*
*1 serving uncooked broccoli heads*

**Mid-afternoon (meal four):**
*1 oz. half-and-half plus 3 large raw eggs (a pre-Rocky practice)*
*1 small protein shake in 6 oz. milk*
*1 or 2 pieces fruit of the day*

**Dinner (meal five):**
*10 oz. low-fat milk*
*8 oz. baked chicken*
*Large vegetable salad*
*Large serving vegetable of the day*
*1 medium baked potato*

**Late evening (meal six):**
*1 medium yogurt mixed with 1 oz. mixed nuts*
*1 small banana*
*1 small protein shake in 6 oz. milk*

Of course, throughout the day I have water by my side and make sure that I drink at least two quarts before the day's end. My favorite vitamin and mineral tablets, Super Spectrim, and a few extra odds and ends are added in the morning and evening. I'm sufficiently fed.

That's it. I know what you're thinking. The guy needs a life, right? The fact is I find pleasure and diversion, joy and fulfillment in an assortment of places and things other than food and eating. It is a strain and displeasure for me to stray from my daily, well-ordered eating pattern to indulge in slurpy, fatty and processed goop. Clean eating works. The affects exceed by a good measure the delights of gourmet indulgences and sugary desserts. I may apply discipline in my diet, but in real life I am a wild and crazy guy.

## A second look

Looking over my figures I'm tossing down about 4,500 calories a day, give or take a couple hundred. That's about right, though it varies; some days I eat more or less, some days I am more or less active. Based on percentage of lean body mass, system efficiency and daily activity level, I estimate that I burn 20 calories a pound. My body weight hovers at 225 pounds: 225 x 20 = 4,500. It's magic.

Should I have the uncontrollable urge to stray from my diet, the rules are strict. No poison. Laree makes the most mouth-watering lasagna in the world, the best chicken cacciatore, Tex-Mex combos and cheesecake. We squeeze those in the lineup where and when we please. We are neither monks nor monkeys. We appreciate what we eat. We are grateful and eat till we're content. The sun goes down at night and rises in the morning, another glorious day. Thank God.

## Habit: The creature from the Black Lagoon

You have an abundance of choices and have chosen consumption beyond your limit to satisfy your cravings of one nature or another. It is fun to eat, after all, and it is the great social pastime. However, eating to the extent that it endangers the quality and length of your life begs contemplation. A light goes on; it's just a bad habit.

Are you one of the numerous overeaters who slid into the habit a long time ago? Most over-consumption can be attributed to a collection of bad habits, which can be controlled or eliminated. That doesn't necessarily reduce the problem to a simple solution; habits are known to have hooks or to be hidden from or denied by the owner. I'm certain that as you established the habits contributing to your largeness so can you modify them to serve your leanness. Habits are like that. Start by identifying them.

Be creative. Add challenge and a subtle ruse: Replace an insufferable habit with any activity—even trivial—that instead contributes to the weight-loss cause.

Hey, got a minute? Meet Lynn.

She's a friend from the gym and this is her story as I've gathered it over the years. It's simple and not incredible, unless you envision what her life might have become had she not identified some bad habits and exchanged them for good.

Every morning at 10, Lynn would leave her office, cross the hall and descend the rear staircase to the vending machines. There she'd insert her coins and select the snack of her choice. "Some choice," she thought, "Snickers, everybody's favorite, gives me a toothache; Cheezios, plastic cheese on stale crackers, sticks to the roof of my mouth; Nutzos, crumbled nuts in a bag, get caught in my throat… and apples. What are the apples doing in the machine?" She always chose the apples because they were natural, nobody else ate them and she didn't want them to go bad. That's the kind of girl Lynn is.

The apple was her snack for other reasons as well. It was nutritious and anybody could see that the other possibilities were probably not; in fact, they looked kinda scary. Lynn had gained useless weight since she took the job in the office, a fact that haunted her. Paperwork, phones and the computer kept her busy, but she seldom moved from the desk and breaks through the day offered the only source of relief. She got into the habit of eating to kill the boredom and hopefully restore her energy. She noticed she'd become sluggish early in the afternoon.

One morning our young lady forgot her change purse and decided to search her car for stray coins. No lost booty in the car, but she found a fresh bottle of water from last night's ball game at the stadium.

She'd parked few blocks down the street that morning to avoid the parking lot traffic. The day was pretty and sunny with billowy clouds that might bring some rain. This was fine with Lynn as the season had been long and dry. The cool breeze off the ocean was the first sign of the coming fall. She drank her water and walked back toward work without haste. "I'll miss the little blue songbirds that leave with the fading summer," she thought, as an exciting gust tousled her hair.

Once at her desk, Lynn sat in a noticeably upright posture. She felt refreshed and the clutter of her desk didn't ruffle her spirits. Brad, with his tanned hands full of office supplies, swooped low as he walked by her desk and said "Hey, Sweetheart," in his Humphrey Bogart voice. He never said hey anything to her before; she laughed and swatted him with a file folder.

Something's up. Lynn was energized, uplifted and hopeful. This was a most unusual afternoon and she wanted to roll into a cartwheel, lately only a fond memory of her early gymnastic training... the good old days.

That evening as she read and fidgeted and prepared her things for work the next morning, her mind drifted and she thought of the day. It was pleasant, and she was stirred. She smiled, realizing the only change was the walk to the car and the bottle of water. And how about that cartwheel? It was amusing that she reviewed her past as if it was so long ago. "Twenty-three, goin' on 40," she grinned to herself.

Impressed by the charge of spirit engendered by the small change in routine, Lynn made a list of personal pet peeves. Four months on the job—a good job with promise—and she was folding in. No real activity and she missed it. She was eating like a bird during the day and a horse at night. Didn't need a nutritionist to tell her that was all wrong. The extra pounds slow a person down, nothing fits and the body, well, she ain't what she used to be. Twenty pounds is brutal—40 soon becomes 60.

Sprawled upon a heap of pillows on her bed, Lynn examined the list once more before turning out the lights. It was a short list and she was both disturbed and thankful. "I'm happy, but I can see the weeds growing in the garden. Time to do some landscaping, girl. Break out the rake." With that she turned out the lights and dreamed of ways to tug out the weeds by the roots and replace them with colorful wildflowers. She was on a mission and felt like she had breathed fresh air into her lungs. "I caught you just in time, you thief," her last thoughts of the night.

She woke up early the next morning with renewed spirits. While her thinking was clear and energy high, she installed three new habits in place of three old, sorry routines.

Number one: Prepare food at home for the workday. Nuts to the vending machine. That morning she filled a water bottle with fresh spring water, packed a brown bag with fruit and hard-boiled eggs. Chicken left over from the night before fit perfectly in the Tupperware. A sense of power rippled through her system as she experienced the control she was exerting in her life. It was unique, a thrill, a freedom, a passion. What took her so long, she wondered, and why aren't more people taking control? Have I been lazy, complacent and unaware? Just fix it. Go forward and don't look back. Make these habits stick.

Number two: Be active and move more when you can at work, for pleasure and refreshment. At break time Lynn took a 15-minute walk around the block, sipped her water and ate some fruit. There's a gym around the corner and she peaked in. During lunch, rather than hang out and gossip with the gang in the lounge, she walked to the gym and ate lunch along the way. She toured the facility, was pleased and thanked the staff member for the free-week trial pass.

Habit number three was to join the gym and reinvent her physical self. The weights weren't the tumbling and high bar that she knew, but they looked fascinating. This would become her new diversion to keep her active and motivated throughout the week. Lynn's plan: two lunch-hour workouts, two during the weekdays after work and one occasionally on the weekends.

"I'm in heaven. Goodbye, fat, and hello, leanness. Take a hike, boredom, and welcome, motivation. Good riddance, guilt and stress, and don't slam the door behind you, ignorance. I'm on my way to the gym."

The story goes on and on. She never misses her workouts and seven friends from work, including Brad, come to the gym regularly. Guess where she got her free-week pass?

## Get a job

Getting back to my stupendous, though unadorned, menu, as I sit at the computer and tap out peculiar notions, I am reminded that it's time for my totally awesome meal number four. Salivating, I'm up and trotting to the kitchen. It's the raw egg combo, Rocky-style, with protein powder and some fruit. Sounds nasty, but I'm aware of the exceptional nutrition the meal supplies and the daring discipline it requires. The contentment is priceless. I don't know what I enjoy more, the discipline or the uncooked eggs going down. You must try it.

I return to my computer invigorated. The sweet flavor of fruit in my mouth and the encouraging sense of good I'm providing myself fills my being: energy restoration, muscle replenishment, and the mind not even slightly twisted with guilt or shame—sterling choices and wise investments, discipline over donuts, persistence over pizza and action over apple pie á la mode. I'm free.

"Guy's warped. And his kitchen is only 20 feet away. What if he had a dysfunctional job that dragged him around the globe or crammed him in a cubicle all day long?" Is that what you say? If I were in the car I'd eat with style: beef jerky, meal replacement bar (MRB), hard-boiled eggs, plenty of water, fruit and nuts. Even the most tyrannical job schedule can be accommodated with will, resourcefulness and your extraordinary goal fixed in your heart and mind.

Early in 2001 I traveled to London, Pittsburgh, Columbus, San Diego, San Francisco and Tulsa over the period of a month. I packed jeans, T-shirts, underwear, pop-top cans of tuna, beef jerky, tubs of protein powder, H2O and MRBs. At one port the aircraft was grounded and we were held overnight. The airlines provided 24 pizzas and cases of canned soda for the passengers and not a crust was left over. I dined on tuna, crackers and low-fat milk. I watched in… what's the right word?… not horror, not disapproval… sorrowful disappointment, I suppose, best describes it, as my flight companions ate and drank that night in the hotel recreation room.

## Food is food is food. I don't think so.

My *Standard Balanced Menu* as listed appears utilitarian because it is. To me it's a sturdy, four-wheel-drive pickup truck without the chrome goodies; roll bar-adorning, mitten-covered night-lights; swaying antennas front and rear, and absurdly oversized tires—It roars. The menu offers variety in taste, smell, texture, mouth appeal and color as well as nutritional value.

Add choice cheeses, sautéed mushrooms and garlic to the hamburger, sprinkle Parmesan on the salad or stir-fry the vegetables, and utility is transformed into gourmet cuisine. Arrange sparingly with flare, add some parsley and you might win the blue ribbon chef award from *Good Housekeeping*.

You can imitate and still be original.

Here's the real deal, brothers and sisters: The plan works. The order, the simplicity, the meal frequency and continuity contribute to one another, and the rewards are generous. Order provides a peace and satisfaction that we yearn for, and simplicity in today's life is an oasis. "Simple" provides freedom from planning and preparing. Draper "simple" means available and inexpensive and less caloric.

Underline this homey little verse: **Meal frequency is the mighty and marvelous dragon slayer.** You receive a continual supply of energy and tissue-building nutrients; your hormones are appropriately stimulated or properly held in check; you never go into a caloric deficit causing the dreaded fat-storing starvation mode and you are never hungry and seldom crave. Did you say you wanted to lose fat and get in shape? Develop and adopt your own version of my standard menu. You've struck it rich.

I've looked over the menus listed in the various dieting books from A to Z. They try to be creative by tweaking the macronutrients here and there, substituting green beans for peas or snapper for tuna. They treat the reader as if he or she had no imagination or resourcefulness, no will or discipline and no capacity to develop any of them. How absurd. We are tough and smart and fascinating.

You be the composer. It's your show... produce, direct, create. Be free. Use the *Standard Balanced Menu* as a template as you calculate the math and food exchanges that work for you. Consider your height, weight, activity, food preferences and realistic goals. Apply your mind—your logic, common sense and instincts—as you strive to match the meal arrangements. Agree not to give up as you juggle your schedule and develop balance and finesse. Keeps you sharp.

For example, you might drop the late meal and lower the caloric intake until your muscle-building program goes into full swing. You can start temporarily with four meals a day if you're accustomed to one plus snacking, still displaying strength and endeavor. Creep up on meat if it gives you the creeps, or do the same with salads or milk. Each day is a lesson as the mistakes, trip-ups and impossibilities foil you and teach you... and it's sometimes frustrating. Frustration is a precursor of inspiration. Oh, and it works. Absolutely.

Just to be sociable, I will outline two menus to accommodate a 1,500 and a 3,000-calorie diet. I call upon your generosity to give me some slack, as I will only approximate the calculations... gives me an opportunity to use my imagination... as you apply yours.

I offer you permission to exercise freedom in your pursuit of weight loss by loosening, not removing, the ropes that bind you. Too tightly restrained and we struggle and quit. With no restraints at all, we wander like children and get lost.

Are you ready? Seat buckles fastened, goggles in place, hands firmly gripping the safety bars; psychologically prepared and fully focused. Let's roll.

# Standard Balanced Menus
## 1,500-Calorie Sample Menu
### Allow approximately three hours between meals.

**Breakfast (meal one):**
*Protein shake (8 oz. nonfat milk, ½ banana, 2 scoops low-carb*
*protein powder)*
*Coffee or tea if desired, and water*
**Meal one total: 323 calories/47 gr protein, 27 gr carbs, 3 gr fat**

**Lunch (meal two):**
*3 oz. grilled lean burger*
*4 oz. 2% cottage cheese*
*Medium tomato*
**Meal two total: 444 calories/54 gr protein, 12 gr carbs, 20 gr fat**

**Snack (meal three):**
*Protein shake (8 oz. nonfat milk, ½ banana, 2 scoops low-carb*
*protein powder)*
**Meal three total: 323 calories/47 gr protein, 27 gr carbs, 3 gr fat**

**Dinner (meal four):**
*4 oz. roasted chicken*
*6 oz. salad with balsalmic vinegar & olive oil*
*6 oz. vegetable of choice, steamed*
**Meal four total: 430 calories/36 gr protein, 28 gr carbs, 19 gr fat**

*Daily totals:*
**1,520 calories/184 grams protein, 94 grams carbs, 45 grams fat**

Okay, so I can't interest you in this week's 1,500-calorie special. Tell ya what I'm gonna do: substitute the hamburger patty with a can of tuna or salmon, bring in turkey meat in place of chicken on meal four and have a small piece of fruit instead of the banana in the shake of mean three. Roasted lamb or brisket make a nice diversion from the roasted chicken and whenever you're feeling wild, add lemon, tea or ice to your water. Life's an adventure. The numbers will fluctuate a tiny bit but who's counting, the IRS?

I strongly advise that you add a high quality time-release vitamin and mineral formula to your food intake, mixed essential fatty acids (EFAs) and a teaspoon of fiber. We don't get enough of these precious gems in our daily treasure chest. Take on a paper route or collect scrap metal for resale to earn the extra bucks if necessary.

Do you think that was high speed, edge-of-your-seat feasting? We now double the calories and macronutrients and experience the creative forces of energy and might as they transform us into reckless molecular activity.

## 3,000-Calorie Sample Menu

### Allow approximately three hours between meals.

### Breakfast (meal one):
*Protein shake (8 oz. low-fat milk, ½ banana, 2 scoops low-carb*
*            protein powder, 1 tsp. peanut butter)*
*Coffee or tea if desired, and water*
*Slice whole wheat toast*
**Meal one total: 505 calories/51 gr protein, 46 gr carbs, 13 gr fat**


### Snack (meal two):
*6 oz. can tuna in water*
*Slice whole wheat*
*Tomato salad (2 tomatoes with balsalmic vinegar and olive oil)*
**Meal two total: 476 calories/44 gr protein, 39 gr carbs, 16 gr fat**


### Lunch (meal three):
*8 oz. low-fat milk*
*4 oz. lean steak*
*4 oz. 2% cottage cheese*
*Medium microwaved red potato*
**Meal three total: 676 calories/73 gr protein, 42 gr carbs, 24 gr fat**

**Snack (meal four):**
*Protein shake (8 oz. nonfat milk, ½ banana, 2 scoops low-carb
protein powder)*
**Meal four total: 323 calories/47 gr protein, 27 gr carbs, 3 gr fat**

**Dinner (meal five):**
*8 oz. low-fat milk*
*6 oz. roasted chicken*
*6 oz. vegetable of choice, steamed*
*6 oz. green salad with balsalmic vinegar and olive oil*
**Meal five total: 535 calories/61 gr protein, 39 gr carbs, 15 gr fat**

**Snack (meal six):**
*8 oz. yogurt topped with ½ banana*
*6 oz. water mixed with 2 scoops low-carb protein powder*
**Meal six total: 441 calories/48 gr protein, 51 gr carbs, 5 gr fat**

*Daily totals:*
**2,956 calories/324 grams protein, 244 grams carbs, 76 grams fat**

The above outlines are as clay is to the sculpture. You have as
much space in which to move as you have creativity. And, please, do
not deny your creativity, that you possess it or have time to implement it. It stirs in all of us and waits for our seeking; it's encouraged by
our beating heart and every breath we take, each moment prompts its
exposure. Neglected creativity is like a beautiful flower in full bloom
with no one to gaze at its glory. Add subtle herbs, a touch ofspice,
some color and behold. Inspiration.

You'll get the hang of it. Later I'll teach you how to zigzag and
dodge the bullet.

---

### Traveling

Going on a road trip? Take a cooler with fruit, vegetables, nonfat milk, tightly wrapped baked potatoes, hard-boiled eggs in their shell. Pack tuna, floods of water, protein powder and your vitamin and minerals. Don't forget your MRBs and beef jerky. Eat out once a day, maybe twice if the pickin's are good. A grocery store rotisserie chicken and a park bench make a nice diversion. If you find yourself on a barren stretch of flat road and you're with your partner and yearn to stretch, take turns pushing your vehicle for a half-hour or so. Just kidding... No, he's not. Or, I don't think so.

---

## Anger cannot be denied. Use it or lose it.

Put order in your life. Start with the basics—your eating and your exercise—and the rest will fall into place. This is the best prescription money can buy, and it's free. Not only free, it comes with incredible benefits.

I feel dumb, tongue-tied and want to come nose-to-nose with the complacent to say, "Read my lips. This works. It works for me and everybody I know and it's going to work for you. Now, do it."

Half the anger we hold is because we're moaning, blaming, neglecting, worrying or resenting. Right? We're denied, misunderstood, obligated and threatened, and 95 percent of it is in our head. I'm telling you (my voice is raised and my face is getting red): Start training today—work out, eat right and adopt it as a way of life. Weight loss will take time. Relax and begin today. Confront yourself under constructive circumstances and see yourself emerge. Don't retreat to the noise of the world: TV, video games or screaming headphones. The fix is certainly not in pizza pie and a pitcher of beer. Get rid of the guilt and size 14 dress (especially you, Bill) and 44 pants (Minerva?). Assert yourself.

## Muscle and fat in balance

What would you like to weigh? Remember, once you're in motion and you've lost the initial casual pounds (excess water, intestinal volume, whatever) and your workouts have taken on momentum, you can plan on losing a pound to two pounds of fat a week. Several variables cause confusion. If you're big-time heavy, you might lose three pounds of fat weekly for an encouraging period without perceptible loss of muscle. If you're working out with weights, which I strongly urge, you will deter the loss of muscle as the weight drops. You might notice that you maintain your body weight (or even gain weight) as you press on in spite of your careful elimination of calories from sugary sources. This apparent stall might present anxiety, but the news is good. You've probably gained valuable muscle mass to complement the shedding of an equal weight in fat. You've gained calorie-burning, vital and dense muscle while burning energy and stored adipose tissue. Way to go!

Such ideal occurrences take place when the differential in fat and muscle is large and one is new to the dieting and weight-training processes. The longer one has been lifting and the more muscle one has in ratio to fat, the less perceptible the muscle growth to the fat loss. Actually, at some point to lose excess body fat, one begins to sacrifice muscle. There are training techniques to overcome these advanced training issues, but they're for another time.

Personally, I hold a safe margin of five to 10 pounds over an ideal, lean weight to maintain strength and energy for tough workouts, fortify my system against injury and illness and feed the muscles all they need for repair and growth. I'm able to train hard and be less critical of subtle muscle tone, which can be distracting. It keeps a smile on my face.

Whatever you do, don't sacrifice muscle by dropping too much weight too fast. Starvation is often the diet of choice, and dieters drop the pounds at any cost. It's not uncommon for the adherents of flimsy low-cal, weight-loss schemes to get rundown, under-muscled, fleshy, weak and irritable. They exhibit signs of compulsiveness and poor judgment. The brain feeds on glucose and they're starving themselves.

# Big Jack

*It was in the spring of '96 when Big Jack stood at the back door of the gym, his patrol car parked and idling next to the dumpster. Garbage was bulging out the half-closed lid and some scraps had escaped and lay conspicuously on the ground. I caught his eye as I walked over with a mighty good explanation for the mess—Darn that new kid I just hired. You know how it is, Officer—and asked how I could be of service on this fine day. He nodded and came right to the point as I inspected the stinky heap with a scowl. "I want to lose the fat and build muscle. Add strength and speed to the body."*

*"You bet. I was just going to clean up this mess, but I'll get to it later. Come on in; let's go inside and take a look around."*

*Being two important men of authority, we got directly to the matter at hand.*

*I said, "We'll make a few adjustments to the Standard Balanced Menu template to suit your calorie needs, Big Jack. You're 5'10", weigh 230 and are a 40-year-old patrol officer. You train at the Y twice a week and are generally active with the job and Little League. You like to eat. The 15-calorie-a-pound calculation sounds about right to me: 230 x 15 = 3,450 calories to keep you happy, Jack... and fat.*

*Your choices include increasing your activity, lowering your caloric intake or an absolutely brilliant combination of the two. Want my advice, what I would do if I were you? Revise your workouts to a three-day-a-week superset program. Increase the intensity 20 percent and take control. Evaluate your menu and plan to limit your daily calorie intake to 3,000 calories by dropping them a hundred a day. Take your time on this challenging backtracking procedure. Feel your way around the job demands, family responsibilities, workouts, sleeping and your well-being, energy and strength. Guessing, I'd say the protein needs to come up and the fat and carbs need to go down. Review my menu as a standard and make sensible changes in your own plan to realistically match it. Fast food goes south. Soda, the junk… you know the drill. Here's one that works for you guys every time: Get those pop-top cans of tuna and pretend they're donuts. You'll get ripped."*

"Can I do this, Dave?" Jack asked. "I'm no kid."

I was staring at his holster and wanted to see his gun. "How's your discipline?" I asked.

"I've got discipline. I'll revive it and follow your advice," he said.

"You can't miss," I said.

"Want to see my gun?" he asked. Nice guy, that Jack.

Jack held on to my words and slowly added walks and sprints at the track as his boys practiced ball. He and the family eventually joined hands and filled an oversized plastic garbage bag with… garbage… from the kitchen cupboards and refrigerator. Nobody missed it, not even the dog.

His upside-down diet was a mess requiring an overhaul and it took a month to sort out the habits, timing and calculations. By early summer the big guy had lost that water bloat and dropped 10 pounds on the scale. His calorie intake decreased from 4,500 to 3,300 and his activity increased as we planned. Thanksgiving arrived, as it always does, and the man in blue was under two. Wendy, his wife who stole workouts on the weekends, discovered bodybuilding was more fun than bowling or cooking. She lost 10 pounds of fat and carried new muscle in her arms and shoulders.

The kids excel in sports today and hope for gym memberships when they turn 13 in 2004. Jack benches 225 for reps at 198 and Wendy has her certificate for personal training. That makes them very good to excellent, but that doesn't make them perfect.

Restores my faith in mankind whose disciplines sometimes wane.

# Not an advertisement—
## It's a public service announcement.

Protein powder supplementation of the health conscious person's diet has been a popular practice for over a half century. "Protein, more protein," was the call of the athlete 50 years ago and his voice is as loud and as clear today. The most popular source of protein powder is milk and its derivatives, partly because of their commercial abundance, but more significantly for their nutritional value: their amino acid constitution and availability to the body for utilization. Whey protein (a milk by-product) has hit the market big time in the last decade and is applauded for its ease of assimilation. Milk casein, long-time champion of protein concentrates, continues to serve mankind in his thirst for the nutritional gold.

The most sought after protein supplement is a blend of the two, as their differing rates of assimilation compliment each other offering both short and long-term tissue-restoring benefits. I believe in supplementation and encourage the use of a good vitamin/mineral and antioxidant formula and a sound protein powder to keep our stores high as we travel the rugged road. My project several years ago (2000) was the development of a custom protein powder for my friends and me. Goal: accentuate the balance of valuable muscle-building and system-repairing ingredients while ignoring the cost. After all, it's for us.

May I introduce you to Bomber Blend, a rare lactose-free mix of the two, blended with significant amounts of B-complex, antioxidants, digestive enzymes, branch-chain (muscle building) amino acids and other key ingredients thoughtfully selected not to crowd out the protein content or destroy the wonderful taste.

We (Laree and I) don't advertise or deal with distributors, so we don't have those monster expenses to pass on to you. I'm very proud of it—it's the talk of the town. You might want to try it.

# Chapter 10

## Jump Higher, Move Faster:
### *"Why?" Reinforced*

And, so, the joyride has begun. You haven't set in concrete the exact details of your weight-loss plan, but an outline is beginning to form. Day by day and page by page the image becomes sharper and more engaging.

I have a friend at the gym who is an athlete and career person, and age has been whispering in her ear. Two years ago when Rita joined the gym and took up weight training, her knees were swelling and aching and her moves on the basketball court were slowing down. She was tough, solid and carried too much weight for a gal hustling up and down a hardwood floor chasing a big ball. We worked together for a few days, and she listened with her whole body. The gym became her training ground.

Rita and I talked recently and recalled the day she began her joy ride, the 35 pounds of extra baggage she lost and how her game improved: "Jumping higher and moving faster and never tiring... I'm stronger, more formidable, relaxed and confident. I was a bully with the extra weight; now I'm a first-class ball player."

I'm wearing a big grin as she reinforces all the practices I preach. "And it wasn't hard to lose the weight. All I had to do was think of the price I pay when I let down my guard. For what? Ice cream and a lot of junk? Am I crazy? My sisters, three of them older than me, are not athletic. I love them, but they're all overweight and often sick.

One has diabetes and high blood pressure, another has had bypass surgery and the oldest is listless. She smokes like a chimney. Sits around like she's expecting cancer."

"It's the couch, the overeating and lack of motivation. No exercise, no support, no desire. They're frightened and I feel sorry for them," Rita said. We stared at each other for a beat. "They won't listen," she continued. She shrugged her shoulders; I shook my head and we resumed our workouts. We were losing our stride and cooling off. We were getting depressed.

I want you to be happy. Life's not perfect; it's frequently disappointing and always a struggle. But, my friend, it has its wonderful moments. You are on your way to losing weight, getting stronger and healthier. What might interfere with your goal? How long will you stick it out? Where will you be should the tough fabric of fortitude unravel? Unfounded negativity. Dismal, yet common, doubts. I proposed them only to point out that they don't concern us. They are for the wearisome and worrisome.

The bittersweet exchange I had with my brave friend highlights the consequences we must consider when a faint tremor of surrender rumbles in our mind. It's the mind that recognizes and cultivates the purposes for losing weight. And, short of legitimate reasons, it's the mind that creates the excuses. You know what to do and why. It's no mystery and it's not rocket science. Never let go or lose sight of your purpose and the rewards. Excuses be condemned.

You who are overweight have real enemies out there that take your breath away: cancers, heart disease, diabetes, high blood pressure, and psychological and social disorders. Take a peek:

• Cancer: It's been observed that either the eating habits that lead to obesity—high-fat, low-fiber diets—or obesity itself is noticeably linked with certain types of cancer.

• Heart disease: Seventy percent of the diagnosed heart disease patients are overweight. A seemingly minor 20-pound weight increase in the average person doubles the risk of heart disease. Strokes and heart attacks only happen to the other guy, right?

• High blood pressure: another common response to an over-weight condition. The over-fat have twice the probability of developing hypertension as someone of normal weight. Heart disease is only a step away.

• Gallbladder disorders: The chances of getting gallstones soars as a person's body weight increases. Those are always a bundle of laughs.

• Diabetes (non-insulin dependent diabetes mellitus (NIDDM) or adult on-set diabetes): This is the disease of the '90s that has the overweight population upside-down. Diabetes is a major killer and we'll talk about it more in another chapter.

• Psychological and social disorders: Rejection, low self-esteem, discrimination, shame and depression claim the lives of many obese people, limiting their joy, creativity, potential and fulfillment. These monsters are henceforth under attack.

Reasonably speaking, whatever your current health, weight, physical and financial environment, you can make significant improvements in your weight-loss and muscle-growth endeavors. It takes willpower, simple foods, basic exercise and determination. Exercise, eat right, for good… make it an everyday affair. If you can put on your jeans, brush your teeth, find the john, stop for a red light, order a pizza and watch the game, you can exercise and eat right for good. Of course, the pizza and the game gotta go.

Tough is good; that's my approach. Alas, tough is a prized trait that is endangered, an irreplaceable excellence lost in the last decades to a brand of disconnected pseudo-toughness that comes from Holly-wood, cartoon heroes, video games, earphones, CDs and the almighty, blazing computer.

The remnant needs to rally and cheer. No habitual splurge days, no fast food in child-size portions, no synthetically sweetened candy or imitation ice cream. A little junk here and a little junk there as long as you don't exceed your minimum daily requirement of precious calories and paltry 50 grams of protein? Treason. These allowances interrupt the discipline-building process and diminish the power of achievement. How does one thrill to the rare sensation of fulfillment while chewing on a mouthful of Gummy Bears? When do we sit down on the hard, cold surface and consider our days without distraction, submission or excuse? Tomorrow?

Today.

# Chapter 11

## Measuring Your Progress:
### *Points of Reference*

It's time we consider the bare facts and gather the raw statistics. How do we go about the delicate task of measuring and what the heck do we measure? Do I gotta?

Again, I expect that a large number of you reading this book are not new to the weight-loss endeavor and are savvy to the various rites of passage to a leaner and stronger body: "Been there, done that" warriors who bear the saber scars and stand considerably taller than before doing battle. I often speak with a familiarity that comes from this assumption. That said, I request room to drift from instructor to gym rat, hoping the granted freedom provides texture for better teaching and learning. I'm with you in the battle—the good fight—and it never ceases.

Tracking your improvement is a very individual and personal procedure. How do you estimate your progress? I, for starters, use the bathroom scale and weigh myself daily. My weight is reasonably stable, yet I do not wish to be surprised by sneaky changes. This tactic works well for me, but scares most people to death. You and the scale should develop your own relationship: Whatever you prefer for whatever reason, fine; just don't let it become more than a tool, a broad guide to serve your purpose.

Weigh yourself at the same time each day with the same apparatus, preferably in the morning on an empty stomach and after elimination, to provide a consistent and accurate reading. A popular recommendation by most weight-control technicians is once a week, but I liken that to driving blindfolded without one's hands on the wheel. (Feel better now? I'm certifiably crazy.) I weigh each morning.

It is important to take into consideration the body is nearly 70-percent water, and fluctuations in water content through the day and throughout the month are normal. These differences are not always predictable and can account for inaccurate estimations that can trip you up. This is one of the reasons I weigh more frequently than commonly suggested; waste or water retention might provide an inaccurate reading on the one day of the week assigned to weighing.

Scary scenario: Sensitive woman weighs herself at 200 pounds when water retention is at an all-time low. Not bad. Two weeks later, after disciplined effort, she weighs herself at 205 when body fluids are at an all-time high. She freaks, poor lady. She failed to consider that her heavy leg and torso workouts have caused a healthy cellular water retention; the intentional high-carb meals according to her carb-loading phase of her intelligent eating plan increased the water in her muscle tissue, and the deliberate increase in daily water intake due to the rising summer temperatures caused abnormal one-day water preservation. Oh, and it's that time of the month. In a single anxious moment when she mounted the deadly scale, her sterling efforts were discounted and the time invested became a cold, hollow space.

Of course, the scale only indicates how much the body weighs. It does not distinguish between body fat and lean body mass (bone and muscle). This indicator, referred to as your percent of body fat, gives a clearer picture of your over-fat condition. I suggest you eventually enter this factor into your calculations to determine more accurately your fat-loss progress. A person might be disappointed that his weight is not dropping, only to discover to his delight that by comparing body fat percentages, his muscle mass increased as body fat decreased. Disappointment—an insufferable state of mind for the hard-working, overweight trainee—is instantly replaced by thankfulness and inspiration. The forward motion continues with reassurance.

The methods for estimating your body fat include underwater weighing, skin-fold calipers, infrared reading and bioelectrical impedance. The body submersion method performed in hospitals and larger weight-loss clinics presents by far the most accurate body fat measurement. The person is lowered into a tank of water where his weight and water displacement are determined. Through a formula based on real weight, submerged weight, displacement and several other related factors, an accurate body-fat-to-lean-muscle ratio is determined.

Skin-fold calipers, like c-clamps, are attached to gathered skin at various sites to assess the percentage of subcutaneous fat. Another formula is applied and a body fat reference is derived. Accuracy depends on the body type of the subject (works better for some than others), water retention, equipment and the tech's skill.

The remaining two methods are done with portable units by a trainer or dietician. They are imprecise and therefore not highly recommended. They can serve as reference points if done for comparison once every six weeks, preferably by the same tech using the same equipment to preserve measuring consistency.

Doctors and dieticians lean toward the Body Mass Index (BMI) for establishing a profile of a person's body fat. I present the formula for calculating your BMI because it is the mainstream standard, though it offers a very loose picture of obesity. It emphasizes the vague, inadequate impression most practitioners accept when analyzing overweight subjects before them. This index indicates that at 6' and 225 pounds, I have a BMI of 31. Thirty qualifies me as obese, yet I am less than 10-percent body fat. Go figure.

Here's the formula to calculate your BMI:

**BMI = *your weight in pounds times 704.5 divided by your height in inches, squared***

The Body Mass Index is interpreted as follows:

**Healthy weight: 19 to 24.9**
**Overweight: 25 to 29.9**
**Obese: 30 and above**

Additionally, the waist measurement is always considered by a weight-loss practitioner when reviewing the BMI. A measurement of 40 inches or more for a man or 35 or more for a woman increases the seriousness of the condition proportionately. It's been observed that those who amass weight around their waists are at a greater risk for developing grave chronic disease than those who hold fat on their hips and buttocks.

Most people long-conscious of their condition can define their overweight level by the way they feel and the difficulty with which they tie their shoelaces; by the way their clothes fit, the notch on the belt and the pinch of flesh at one or two all-too-familiar sites. The mirror is an honest device that knows not how to lie, cannot be bribed and has no sense of humor. Cruel and pitiless are the words often used to describe its silent stares.

It's not uncommon to gain muscle density as you lose fat and, therefore, see no change in body weight. A comparison of muscle measurements can often validate real training progress, replacing frustration with inspiration to press on. Recording measurements of five primary body areas (chest, waist, hips, arms and thighs) for reference is not a bad idea. I dare you.

## Take five

I pause as I write and realize I'm reluctant to move on without shoring up your courage. Measurements, comparisons, gauging and uncovering the naked truth can be dangerous. They are not—neither one nor all together—an absolute indicator of the real progress you are making. I contend that your advancement is continual as you apply yourself with diligence and appropriate intensity to the precepts and practices offered in this book.

Once you are in motion and time has been invested, chemical changes are taking place that are not visible. Hormonal and enzymatic balances responsible for muscle growth, fat loss and body harmony are under transformation, and their benefits are not always externally evident. Internal fortification is in progress. As the farmer accepts patiently the natural laws, so must we. There are seasons for planting. There are seasons for harvesting, and there are seasons that are slow to produce. Be faithful. Soon your storehouse will overflow.

Not all growth is measurable with a yardstick or a scale. How do you weigh perseverance? Can you take a tape to discipline or calipers to ingrained determination? It is these shapely and well-defined appendages of the spirit and mind that carry you toward your goals. There is a fine cooperation between the weight you lose and the character you gain, the tone of your muscles and the tenor of your fortitude. Always the latter will precede the former.

I accept that advancement can be estimated by the success with which one forestalls diminishing; that is, not by how much a person goes forword, but how little a person goes backward. There comes a time in age when forward is not an option; preventing the rate of backward descent is, always.

The ups and downs are inevitable. None of you are exempt. Those who give up cannot expect the highs to be too high. They— the quitters—had better adjust to the length, width and duration of those relentless lows.

Persistence overpowers lagging endurance. Desire outweighs defeat. Courage rules. Success is in the achieving that never quite ends.

# Chapter 12

## The Bane of Women:
### *Menopause & Weight Gain*

The playing field has become for many a battleground. Earlier I sketched a rough figure of an overburdened society beset with weakening influences and misguided thinking. Review of the last 50 years confirms that a growing number of men and women have gained weight and lost health, and have become soft, less active, dispirited and less creative.

The trouble has been confronted and its source disclosed, a resolution decided and the plan of action forthcoming. You and I are fixing the problem and that's that.

Man has his hands full. He envisions himself as lifting the load, moving the earth, leading the land, protecting its borders, making touchdowns and being a cowboy.

You'd think a strong physique would naturally accompany his brawny functions, yet he is bundled in fat and hides behind his prodigious girth instead. He has a tough job to do and a tough image to follow.

The struggle for women to achieve and maintain a lean and strong figure is doubly hard, and the image expected of her is twice as great. It behooves you, men, to read this chapter to better understand yourself and more fully appreciate your partners and the unfair battle they fight.

The calamity of image is obvious. Women are expected to look vaguely like the under-nourished models that parade across the gilded stage of life. Queens of fashion are 20ish, tall and slender and flaw-lessly made up; they are ravishing, rare and temporary. The average woman is twice her age, eats and works and chases kids around the house. I cannot dismiss the brutal power that image exerts in the lives of my female friends and the pleasure or pain it brings in the course of their days. It must be tedious, distracting and downright infuriating to be under the gaze of the whole world, the all-too-familiar once-over that comes with the feminine form. And to make matters worse, man—woman's greatest admirer—immaculately executes his role, the big gawking dope.

Men, be thankful. Take nothing for granted. There is no monthly cycle that you need to suffer with its discomfort, physical inconvenience, water retention, cravings, malaise, fatigue, aching and hormonal havoc.

I'll pass on squats and deadlifts this week, guys.

Man is spared the dubious privilege of bearing children and enduring pregnancy and the trauma to which the body is subjected: stretched, pushed, pulled, excruciated and consumed. Thank God, but what a job.

And then there is undeniably the most popular and delightful of women's crosses, the inevitable period of menopause that seems to go on forever and offers one unpredictable day after another. The accompanying hormonal changes dictate her chemistry, state of physical and mental health, body shape and fat retention. Few women slip by unscathed; few women understand the process and most women are victims of an undefined opponent.

Needless to say, I, the Blond Bomber from the '60s, Mr. America and Mr. Universe, know all about menopause. Claiming your confidence and having conferred with a few female experts, I attempt to illuminate the darkness of menopause and the expanded influence it has on your female existence. According to rusty-yet-common thought, the mid-life transition is expected to last two to four years, commencing with the retreat of menstrual cycles. While this is true of the extreme changes, menopause is surrounded by possibly 20 years of hormonal preparation and alteration. This time span ranging from ages 35 to 55—one quarter of life—is known as perimenopause.

Estrogen is the primary female hormone made and secreted by the ovaries and responsible for the stimulation of female secondary sex characteristics and the growth and maintenance of the reproductive system. Menopause, a natural transition, involves the diminishing of the ovaries' fertilizing activity and is accompanied by a decrease in estrogen production. The body detects mild losses of estrogen during the perimenopausal years and comes to the aid of the ovaries to manufacture the vital hormone. The most efficient place for estrogen production is in the fat cells. They increase in number, size and fat-storing efficiency. This sounds like a bad dream, but it's the body's faithful care for your menopausal health.

The fat cells in your midsection are the first to grow and grow the largest because they are better constructed for the manufacture of estrogen than the fat cells in your hips, buttocks and thighs. How many of you gals at 35 realize you are currently in the business of assembly line fat-cell production and business is booming? Your fat cells are in overdrive turning out estrogen that counters the early indicators of the menopausal blues: hot flashes, mood swings, cramping, aching, swelling and uneasy sleep.

Fine. Ignorant of the natural protective devices of the body, you diet and your efforts to combat the weight gain fail. Bummed, bothered and bewildered, you give up only to try again, another diet that worked like gangbusters last year. No good. Moping inactivity, of course, is the common companion of failed diets—leading to increased body fat and frustration. Now sedentary, the body is released of its need for muscle and gives up at least half a pound of its precious inventory each year and a minimum of two pounds of fat replaces the stock. In the 10 years between ages 35 and 45 you lose five pounds of fat-burning, life-supporting muscle and gain 20 pounds of the cumbersome fat stuff. Chances are very good that you've lost calcium and you're staring osteoporosis in the eye.

Your plan to deal with menopause at any stage is to recognize and accept the transition as a part of your being and know that your healthy approach will minimize its draining affects. Eat right and exercise with an accent on exercise. Aerobics serve to strengthen the cardio-respiratory system and encourage the manufacture of fat-releasing enzymes that trigger the emptying of stored fat into the blood-stream for energy. But aerobics alone will not build muscle; strength training needs to be included. Muscle-building resistance exercise stimulates fat burning and the new muscle cells contribute 25 percent to estrogen manufacture, thus liberating the fat cells of the entire hormone-subsidizing project. They can shrink in size without compromising estrogen production.

It's time to regain what you lost of the priceless sinewy mass that holds you together, that moves boxes to the attic, couches across the living room and carries your toned body smoothly and steadily up hills and mountains. Instead of losing muscle mass from this day forward, gain it and shape it and encourage it to work for you. It takes time and work to build the stuff, but muscle doesn't just sit there and look swell. Muscle burns fat for you while you sleep and eat. And acquiring this valuable resource is not grim labor; it's an invigorating diversion with expression, intensity and powerful life-giving rewards.

Be strong and courageous. Along with the epidemic overweight condition is the decline in physical strength. Surveys show that a quarter of the female population 40 to 55 have difficulty with every-day activities: climbing stairs, walking the mall or lugging packages. Balancing and flexibility are lost early due to decreased activity and healthy nerve and muscle interplay. Increased body fat, vanishing muscle and lost strength are a trio dragging you to disaster. Look around; the gruesome threesome is real, insidious and heading this way. You can stave off the nasty combination by exercising, starting today. It works for all ages.

Women, who among you—and be aware that we're all watch-ing and listening—are planning to put a comprehensive exercise scheme in motion? Are you going to sit there passively as your life is abbreviated? Could you stare at a wound as it bled without applying pressure to stop the leaking life?

Start with an hour this week… 10 minutes a day and take Sun-day off. Double it by the end of the month and take two days off. Anything goes… get moving, walk, walk and jog, walk with a weighted pack on your back, carry small hand weights and walk up steep hills or climb stairs wherever they can be found along the way. Move with determination and physical force as you break walking barriers. You're not going to give in to weakness and physical deterioration, nor fat nor the foolishness that attends these unacceptable conditions. You have a heart that beats and blood that moves warmly through your veins and arteries, a mind that thinks and creates and imagines, and it's all yours... feelings that are deep and wide and known only to you.

What's so funny? Right now it's time to meditate on and embrace with love and affection a set of crunches and a set of leg raises. Hop to it, girls.

# Female Facts

While digging around the literature focused on women and their unique concerns, I came across some dandy insight you might find interesting.

Polycystic Ovary Syndrome (PCOS) is an unhappy condition where excess testosterone is secreted in a female, and secondary male characteristics develop: facial hair, bulkiness, and Tomboy tendencies. This unwelcome deviation can sometimes be attributed to improper protein, carbohydrate or fat intake and easily adjusted by dietary measures. If you know a young lady who would rather change the oil in her car or wear work boots and carpenter's pants instead of shopping for designer cloths at the mall, give her the scoop. Dietary changes might very well accentuate the lady within.

Testosterone is the hormone of choice for men, but women need to recognize the important role the predominantly male hormone plays in their system as well. Contrary to PCOS, improper (low) levels of the signaling mechanism can lead to fatigue, depression and loss of muscle. Next visit to your gynecologist have a blood test and take a look at your hormonal balance. You owe it to yourself.

# Scientists at work

Researchers do the darndest things. One day, when things were dull in the laboratory, they took samples of fat cells from the buttocks of nearby men and women. Here's what they found:

• A woman's fat cell is larger than a man's—five times larger.

• Her fat cells have at least twice the fat-storing enzymes as a man's.

• Female fat cells have half the fat-releasing enzymes as a male's.

• Of course, woman's propensity to hold fat is attributed to her child-bearing and nurturing function.

• Furthermore, other studies prove that man has a greater percentage of muscle mass and burns fat more efficiently. Neat, but it catches up with the ole boy, because:

• Women live eight to 10 percent longer lives, and if there's a famine, men are the first to go.

# Chapter 13

## Facts & Fiction:
*Helpful Knowledge & Understanding*

You've been hanging on my every word and I commend you. Brenda, would you, please, nudge the lady next to you who's snoring like a lumberjack and sliding down in her seat? Thanks.

I'm going to pass out some random tips and hints, facts and fallacies to fill in the gaping holes I tend to dig.

## Act I, Scene I:
## Serotonin, Endorphins, Dopamine

The body is a grand theater presenting an intense play composed of complex plots and subplots. A cast of macronutrients—the famous protein, infamous fat and beloved carbohydrate—and the cast of supporting characters, the micronutrients—vitamins, minerals and lesser-known metabolites—share the starring roles. Set with the backdrop of vivid and colorful hormones, the sweeping true-life story unfolds. Creativity and intelligent management are exhibited by the neurotransmitters busy in the brain, setting the mood, temper, energy and appeal of each moment after splendid moment.

Neurotransmitters, talented co-workers numbering more than 500, are assigned irreplaceable tasks under the leadership of an artistic team comprised of four popular directors: the serotonin, endorphins, dopamine and norepinephrine. The stage is set for high drama.

Neurotransmitters are highly complex and interactive chemicals that control brain responses: mood, food craving, sexual excitement, mental acuity, motivation, energy, drowsiness and so on. Our mental and emotional health depends upon the proper balance of these transmitters and they are directly related to the interactivity of hormones, smart exercise, right food intake, exposure to sunlight and more.

The endorphins are associated with pain killing and the increased sense of well-being during intense exercise. Dopamine and norepinephrine assist in mental productivity and clarity.

Serotonin is the neuro-substance closely related to mood and mind comfort and promotes the feeling of satiety, or fullness. Particularly interesting is high-carbohydrate (high-sugar) foods and their upward affect on insulin, which increases the levels of serotonin and thereby improves feelings of well-being. It follows that the not-un-common experience of depression or anxiety is accompanied by a yearning for carbohydrate-rich foods. You have a craving for sugar not necessarily based on hunger but the need to satisfy a chemical imbalance—the shortage of serotonin—in your brain chemicals.

*Excessive* presence of this neurotransmitter, on the other hand, decreases energy and mental sharpness, causing fatigue and drowsiness. High insulin plays havoc with serotonin, taking sugar addicts on the rollercoaster ride that defines their life.

Serotonin levels drop as estrogen levels decrease accounting for the cravings women deal with in perimenopausal and premenstrual phases of their lives.

The fix to hormonal imbalance is regular exercise and the avoidance of over-consumption by eating smaller, balanced meals more frequently throughout the day. These same habits provide the regulated and beneficial presence of neurotransmitters in the brain. And, mysteriously, weight control and appetite suppression are accomplished by following the same scheme. General health substantially improves and everything you touch turns to gold.

Complex in the explaining, easy in the achievement: Exercise and eat right for good.

## Protein

I emphasize high-protein ingestion for more than one reason, or two. Not only do muscles require this marvelous ingredient to repair and grow, but also three-quarters of the solids in the body—hair, skin, bones, etc.—are comprised of proteins. Specific amino acid combinations act as signaling molecules and serve as part of the neuromuscular system and, not unlike neurotransmitter activity, contribute to how we feel.

There are unending complex variables that determine the assimilation of, and need for, protein in all its amino acid combinations and concentrations: the mass of the system, its relative health and efficiency, general activity level, body composition (muscle to fat ratio), protein digestibility, stress and other factors, such as gender and age. I seek to be protein-rich, not due to greed but efficacy.

I want to remind you that your plan is to lose weight healthfully with a strong grip on life. It calls for you to build muscle and grow in vigor and might. You are not committing to a 12-week program to lose 24 or 48 pounds of anything, whether it's fat, muscle, hair, skin or bone... heart or soul. You're here to add muscle and lose fat. It is clear that increased blood levels of amino acids improve protein synthesis (muscle growth) in skeletal muscles. Relax. You will not become a bonehead.

You're committed for good, one day at a time. What you lose is gone; what you gain is here to stay. The premise is brilliant, and it calls for quality protein. At varying levels man is always engaged in restoring and building muscle. The need for protein for auxiliary fuel and amino acids for muscle development and system support are significantly greater for those who exercise and assume a weight-loss program.

It has been rumored that high protein intake is toxic and harmful to the system. These claims are an exaggeration and without documentation. (I have just alienated a mob of doctors now preparing for my tar and feathering – I hate that – who insist my statement is false.) There is no such negative evidence when dealing with healthy subjects. Extraordinary amounts of protein ingested over an extended period of time "might" adversely affect the kidneys; only if pre-existing conditions exist are precautions advised. See your doctor if suspicious.

We may also hear and read from various vague sources that a

high protein intake leaches calcium from the bones. Scary generalization. While it's true that demineralization accompanies a high protein meal (evident in high mineral content found in urine), it is not proven in any study that a regular muscle building, high protein intake leads to long-term mineral deficiency. Calcium and other minerals alone do not account for bone strength; there is a significant protein matrix upon which bones, cartilage and ligaments depend. Further, there is evidence that older folks on high protein diets have fewer stress factors than those whose intake is low. Listen to your mom and drink your milk. Take your supplements.

A protein-rich diet is essential in your journey to lose fat, strengthen your body and improve your health. Don't worry. An overabundance of protein will only lead to protein oxidation, a condition that some researchers speculate will initiate "anabolic drive" or accelerated protein synthesis. That's always been my logic and theory. Yours, too?

The daily protein intake suggested in the United States Recommended Daily Allowances (USRDA) and, therefore, by most nutritionists, is barely sufficient for survival. Is that what you have in mind for you and your family, just enough to get by? Why, certainly, you say, my family and I are not greedy people. Waiter, we'll have hardly enough protein. And while you're at it, please skimp on the vitamins and minerals.

If you get stingy with your protein, the amino acid levels drop, non-essential functions are compromised and skeletal muscle protein synthesis falls to a minimum. Glutamine, a primary muscle component, is robbed from the cells to fuel the hungry immune system. Similar amino acid swaps cripple the body's ability to cope with the stress and tissue damage induced by the heavy load of the tough life. Researchers fear that man is actually predisposed to illness because of the limited protein reserve that accompanies the U.S. Department of Agriculture (USDA) and the U.S. Department of Health and Human Services' RDA.

The research done to establish the RDA figures are old and outdated, yet they remain on the books like barnacles on a rusted, sunken enemy destroyer. They were formulated to give the general public an indication of the minimum allowance of micro- and macronutrients for sustaining life—preventing starvation—under minimal life stress. The researchers weren't considering the demands of living as we know them today nor were they up to speed with hormonal complexities, high-performance expectations, disease, aging and life extension.

Recognized as a major player in stamina and sustenance, the active and strong seek protein from its primary sources: meat, fish, poultry, eggs and milk products. There protein in all its sub-elements—amino acids—is found in generous supply. Nuts, beans, grains and legumes contain valuable protein also, but in limited proportions. And our wonderful, life-supporting, living vegetables and fruits, though high in vitamins and minerals, offer only a few aminos to the high performer's stock.

In closing, I offer you the following sage advice: Wallow in protein. Slather it on in great gobs. Stuff it into your mattress. Hide it under the floorboards. Gulp it when they're not watching. Eat protein and fly with the eagles.

## Ya gotta eat

Another important point I want to underscore while I have your undivided attention: Don't starve yourself.

Some doctors might prescribe a radically low intake of balanced foods or a liquid diet for particular patients, but these are exceptions and careful supervision is required.

Impatient dieters with compulsive tendencies often set themselves up for failure by limiting their calorie consumption to some absurdly low number far below their basal metabolism, and the body instinctively reacts as if it was being starved. It slows down the metabolism to spare the calories and begins to store them as fat. Gets worse: Amino acids, a very efficient fuel source, are burned to keep you trudging along. Stop there. Amino acids are protein. Muscle is protein. Get your greedy mitts off my muscle.

Low blood sugar accompanies this low-calorie practice and the brain finds itself short of its primary fuel, glucose. At best, if calories are sufficient to keep you going, you'll exhibit irritability, argumentativeness, apathy and lethargy. Big trouble can follow: blurry vision, jitters, fainting, coma and, in rare instances, death.

Chronic and extreme dieters who display these tendencies need to have their noses tweaked. They are overly emotional, obsessed with food and quick to eat excessively when they near the edge. Listen to me for a second. Give exercise a chance. Barbells beat the binging blues.

One more thing: After a good night's sleep—or even eight hours of tossing and turning—you must feed yourself to avoid all the aforementioned trouble. Break the fast as the word "breakfast" indicates. I'm not hungry in the morning, and I don't want to fuss. This is when a tasty and efficient protein powder comes in handy. I make up a smoothie with low-fat milk, fruit, ice and two or three scoops of protein powder—a nutritious, well-balanced meal to serve me fuel and system-satisfying ingredients till mid-morning.

## "There is no magic pill."
### *1649, a year before the fall of the Empire*

First came an announcement from the great balcony that rose on monumental columns of gray stone high above the crowds; a dour figure dressed in thick black fabric bellowed through a cone-shaped device, his voice deep as a pit, as dark, as final, "There is no magic pill." Cold steel silence pierced the hearts. No one moved, dejection too heavy a burden. "There is no magic pill." Clouds moved, swift and ominous, as if roused by the declaration, murderous in its conclusiveness.

One by one the shadowy horde dispersed. "They promised… they pledged, they swore a better way: a pill to burn fat, to lose weight, build muscle and strength and add years to fleeting life. They said yes." The moon rose clear and bright, the stars sparkled, the breeze murmured; night birds sang, the jasmine breathed its lovely fragrance but no one noticed. Beauty failed to stir them. "What will we do?"

We're not among the sorry masses whose backs are without muscle and whose characters know no strength. Hard work and discipline define our journey, challenge and fulfillment our joy. The magic pill—a mix of deception and imagination—is offered on late night infomercials and static-filled radio stations along with fat-burning, muscle-building, waist-trimming electronic impulse devices (give me a break) as a means to the same end, make someone bucks and give the needy false hope. May they wake up tomorrow morning layered with genuine blubber.

Don't turn the page yet, partner in good deeds and practitioner of worthy causes. We are not without our innocent little helpers and honest tiny friends. There are friendly thermogenics; pill or liquid concoctions whose ingredients tend to raise the body's temperature by increasing its activity (a form of metabolic enhancement), thus requiring stored calories to lower the body's artificial temperature increase. Stimulants in the form of caffeine and ephedrine raise the bodily activity and heat, and add to one's training outut on the gym floor. Zoom-zoom. Energy and endurance take a step forward. Cooperating with ingredients are chromium (a mineral) and L-carnitine (a bio-active metabolite), each a factor in transporting blood sugar and fat, respectively, into the cells for energy efficiency—a win-win situation, as the corporate hip always say. As intended, thermogenics appear to be as safe as strong coffee, given no pre-existing heart conditions— if concerned, check with your doc. Taken by the jar they are troublesome.

Several popular mainstream products include Twin Labs Ripped Fuel Caps, American Bodybuilding Products Ripped Force and Hydroxycut. Used before a workout they will smoothly increase energy for the duration of the training session while calling upon blood lipids and blood sugar for fuel. Appetite blunting is not uncommon. As always, attend to your pre-workout fuel stores and post-workout replenishing with a blended protein shake. If you decide to try them, take only as indicated by the manufacturer and only when you work out. Be wise.

## Stress

As a match can ignite a campfire to produce warmth and light, or cook food and boil water, so can it set a forest ablaze and destroy nature and wildlife. Stress is similar in that it has both creative and destructive tendencies. Stress in man signals an emergency condition and his whole body chemistry goes into a survival mode. The chemistry involved is extensive and fascinating. The point is that stress is good and alerts and prepares man to save his life. Every athlete, public speaker and actor will underline the positive role stress plays in preparing him or her for an enthusiastic and bright performance.

Another time, as the days and weeks go by, the stress of daily life not going man's way causes turmoil in his mind, emotions and physical body. This, too, is interesting and complex, and affects his life dramatically. The difference is this stress is bad and, you might say, slowly kills him. The indirect causes can be psychogenic and be manifest in destructive behavior. These might be reflected in eating disorders, anorexia, bulimia or over-consumption.

Stress can take its toll on the body by continually inducing disturbances in chemistry. Excess acid in the stomach is just one painful condition, which, unchecked, might develop into ulcers or chronic digestive problems. Stress interferes with sleep, which in turn interferes with recovery, energy and the beneficial release of growth hormone, mankind's particularly good friend.

Ironically, stress too often prevents our going to the gym or taking precious time to exercise when it is the exercise that reduces stress and wholesomely redirects the animal to do good deeds. And, dear friend, you know we eat most of the time because we're stressed, not because we're hungry. The vicious cycle must be willfully interrupted by you for your sake, ASAP or sooner. Be gentle with yourself and take a stick to stress.

The release of cortisol, the primary stress hormone, is triggered by stress. The main characteristic of cortisol is that it stimulates catabolism or the breakdown of muscle into fuel. Again, the body under stress is told to survive at all cost, the repair of muscle tissue is halted and it is instead used as very expensive fuel for more important tasks: feeding the brain, preserving the heart and other principal life-sustaining functions. Time for Stress Management 1A.

We've considered these observations for a long time and it's good to be reminded that, though moderate levels of stress are safe and often beneficial, excessive, modern-day stress is destructive and is to be avoided by every means and trick available. Here's something you might not know: A report by a senior scientist, Dr. Pamela Peeke, formerly with the National Health Institute, informs us that "There are special receptors on the fat cells deep inside the abdomen which are specifically intended to hook up with the stress hormone... and the stress hormone stimulates them to accept fat." The body is predisposed to store fat for those times when it is under stress and engages the "flight or fight" defense mechanism. Since the brain can't distinguish survival stress from chronic, daily stress, anyone who experiences stress overload will store more fat. Oh, boy.

Dr. Peeke, a very cool individual, I gather, says that relaxation and other forms of passive stress management are not enough to stem stress and its ravages. The best way to block stress hormones is through beta-endorphin, a neurotransmitter produced during exercise. "Weight lifting on a routine basis… at least twice weekly vigorously for 30 to 40 minutes… for both men and women is really the key," Peeke says. She went on to say that protein from lean sources was important and people should avoid starches (sugars). Redirecting the stress at the gym works wonders.

It really gets crazy when we consider the role stress plays in stimulating or suppressing certain hormones responsible for muscle growth or fat storage. Hitting the workouts eliminates the cascade of trouble stress causes and precludes the need to read volumes on the subject. That's the Cheap Draper Solution (CDS); works every time.

## Essential fatty acids

The three-letter word "fat" has caused more trouble in the world than a barrel of hungry monkeys. The mere formation of the proper one-syllable noun on our lips is disturbing, its sound to our ear abrasive and the thought of it repugnant. Dietary fat is condemned like a criminal, and we face the sentencing. We find upon close examination that the terribly uncouth character comes in all shapes and sizes depending on its molecular structure and contrary to popular opinion, most fat (except for the slabs covering our bodies) is very, very good. It has a complex variety of functions, properties and distinctions. It supports us liberally and a moderate consumption of good dietary fat promises us a long and healthy life.

Fat serves to support, protect, shape and cushion the body, internally and externally. It is necessary for the absorption of the fat-soluble vitamins A, D, E and K, and very low-fat diets disrupt their absorption. The health of the immune system is largely dependent upon fat consumption, moderate fat intake proving more beneficial than low-fat intake.

Our lives depend on fats that our bodies do not produce. These are called essential fatty acids (EFAs) and must be supplied through the diet. Hormone-like compounds called prostaglandins are synthesized from EFAs and control an endless string of crucial, moment-to-moment life functions including blood pressure, blood clotting, nerve impulses, insulin sensitivity and hormone responses. EFAs transport oxygen in a long journey from the lungs to the cells, increase stamina, speed healing, improve the general feeling of well-being, give lustrous health to the skin and hair; they aid in the prevention of arthritis, and lower cholesterol and triglycerides. They are essential for rebuilding and producing new cells. Without them our health is drastically compromised, we degenerate and we die.

Quickly, two basic categories of EFAs that you need to know:

First, Omega-3 (w3) includes alpha-linolenic acid (LNA) found in meat, fish, fish oil, and certain superunsaturated vegetable oils such as canola, olive and particularly flaxseed oil.

Next, Omega-6 (w6) includes linoleic (LA) and gama-linolenic acids (GLA) found in raw nuts, seeds, legumes, sesame and soybean oil and especially safflower oil. Hemp oil is a first rate source of both Omega 3 and Omega 6 EFAs. More and more research is being done on conjugated linoleic acid, or CLA, a natural derivative of linoleic acid, which is revealing fat reducing, muscle building qualities. The magic bullet?

These oils are sensitive to heat, light and oxygen and extreme care is required in maintaining their wholeness and activity. Though they are available in our diets, as are all essential nutrients, because of their instability and because of their vital importance, I highly recommend that they be added as a supplement. Some people mix the oils in protein drinks or salad dressing. I gulp down a smart blend of flaxseed, safflower and hemp oil twice a day to assure a healthy ratio of all the EFAs available to splendidly direct the show. They come in capsules, kids.

Earmark this page to remind you of the importance of EFAs and the effort you must put forth to gain them in your diet. You see, EFAs ingested in sufficient levels (12 to 15 percent of total calorie intake) increase the rate of metabolic reactions in our body, thereby burning more fat into energy and waste... bottom line, fat burning and excess weight loss. Oh, my.

Fat is, or was designed to be, an efficient fuel for the body. Recently, as we have dramatically altered our existence, the fuel of choice has shifted to sugar, another wrong choice by man. Compelled by greed he has put forth the deception that carbohydrate is needed as the chief source of energy. There are big profits in sugar; it's cheap and easy to sell.

Thus, modern man has altered his fat metabolism and has become a hyperglycemic sugar burner, consequently ridden with ailments and imbalances. He's up and down with the glucose fluctuations, hormones jump about like crickets in mid-summer, insulin can't accommodate his capricious appetites; sugar storage is saturated and the fat is generously deposited. Obesity, heart disease, diabetes and hyper- and hypoglycemia bully our lives.

## Cholesterol

Anyone with a pulse has heard the horror stories about cholesterol. In fact, we are led to believe that cholesterol is one of the evils responsible for the pause or cessation of that pulse when we least expect it. Most of the medical world says cholesterol attaches itself to our artery walls, hardens them, restricts them, stops the flow of blood and we suffer angina, occlusions, embolisms and gangrene; and, cholesterol goes hand in hand with heart disease and obesity. Let me spend a dime of your time and clear the air, or at least attempt to thin the fog. Though definite problems with cholesterol arise in modern societies, there is a side to this hard, waxy lipid upon which the sun does shine.

Cholesterol is essential for our health. Take a look:

• Cholesterol is needed within the cells to regulate the ever-changing fluidity of cellular membranes.

   • Sex hormones (steroid hormones) are made for us by cholesterol.

   • Other vital hormones that suppress inflammation, assist in survival energy surges and regulate water retention are made by the poor undervalued lipid, cholesterol.

• Vitamin D, the sunshine vitamin necessary for the metabolism of calcium and phosphorous, is made from cholesterol.

• Bile acids, integral in the digestion and absorption of fats, oils and fat-soluble vitamins are derived from cholesterol.

• We find cholesterol secreted by glands in the skin covering and protecting it from the ravages of external trauma (water, sun, wind) and infection.

• Cholesterol drags itself to our relief as an anti-oxidant when our store of vitamin and mineral antioxidants is low. Our little, misunderstood hero.

We would have fewer problems with cholesterol if we ate right and exercised. Even those with a genetic predisposition to cholesterol harms would do a lot better. Our bodies manufacture cholesterol quite readily and are pressed to make an abundance of the ingredient when we consume excess calories, particularly from sugars and saturated fats. Stress, too, triggers the body to make more cholesterol because it is a precursor of stress hormones. Stress and excess calories from junk foods are gremlins of the modern world over which we have control. Exercise and eat right regularly to reduce the high-cholesterol scares… and many more.

A peculiarity of cholesterol that adds to its special handling is that the body can make it, but cannot break it down, as it can sugars, fatty acids and proteins. It can only be eliminated efficiently through the stool, and then only if adequate fiber is present in the diet. Add fiber to your smart eating.

We are buried in research about cholesterol and different schools of thought are emerging. Some say the human being is not designed to metabolize large amounts of dietary cholesterol, or he is not equipped to regulate its distribution, or his cholesterol-removing fiber is far too low. Thus, cholesterol contributes to the widespread disease of arteriosclerosis—hardening of the arteries.

I'm a meat eater who includes eggs and dairy, as well as fruits and vegetables in his menu and don't hesitate recommending the diet to you. My total cholesterol level hovers at 132 year after year. Two out of 10 might have to be cautious of their dietary cholesterol, but is that a hard truth if they exercise and bring in fiber and the micronutrients that provide balance and efficacy in the system?

I lean toward the findings of those stimulating scientists who point out that "cholesterol problems" can be avoided or resolved by supplying the body with adequate vitamins and minerals often deficient in those foods that are high in protein. To enjoy the muscle-building, fat-burning benefits of protein-rich foods, bring in the micronutrients and accessory ingredients that assist their metabolism, absorption, transportation and eventual healthy elimination. The addition of certain micronutrients (vitamins C, B3, and minerals calcium, zinc, copper and chromium) plus omega-3 EFAs, fiber and regular exercise diminish damaging lipid levels, reduce stress and make you strong—a prescription for the defense against and reversal of cardio vascular disease and obesity. Some of these factors can be derived from our daily diet, but not in the quantities we require. Be prepared to supplement your food intake.

I'm not a political troublemaker or a health food activist, yet I can't ignore some distinct fallacies in the market place and in the medical community that inhibit our development. The news and advertising media have us convinced that the low fat and cholesterol free diet is an answer to the broad base of health problems. Those diets, in fact, might indirectly lead to health problems far worse than holding too many extra pounds, including suicide (serotonin uptake in the brain is inhibited due to lack of cholesterol and depression and aggressive behavior go unchecked) and cancer (disease-fighting antioxidant uptake in the system is suppressed due to lack of cholesterol).

We are also encouraged to use cholesterol-free margarines as a butter substitute only to find that they typically contain the most dangerous oils in the refrigerator. "Cholesterol free" is a goldmine to the packagers of modern foods. Let's keep our eyes open.

Two-time Nobel Prize-winning Dr. Linus Pauling and his associate, Dr. Matthias Rath, put forth the theory that the lack of vitamin C in the body is responsible for cardio vascular disease, thickening arteries, high blood pressure and a cascade of problems that have us suffering in the far corners of our system. The comprehensive study centering on a single magnificent micronutrient, vitamin C, upset a medical community that was long targeting cholesterol as the villain. Support was anemic. Printing of the report in well-read and prestigious journals was at first approved and later rejected. Politics and economics rose above the head of the Nobel Prize winner and we wait for the sun to shine and the mist to evaporate. Don't wait for science to sign the bottom line to your contract for an extended and prosperous life. Be aware, look, listen and act. Exercise and eat right regularly.

## Complex hang-ups

Eating and the emotions can be interwoven, and the doctors studying eating disorders and treating suffering patients have their hands full. I believe the readers of this book are at least aware that these complex conditions exist if not what to do to combat them. What can we do, here and now, if these subtle conditions afflict you?

I know you have fantastic potential. You can do extraordinary things with the information and conversation you're getting in these thin pages. You've already started by confronting yourself with the challenges I've put forth. You're considering what I say and its validity and appeal. What about muscle building and my references to weight training, protein and the inevitable loss of fat through an honest and admirable way of life? It works. This I know for sure.

Treat what I say less like cold, hard facts that are onerous in the thought and ponderous in the doing. Is that how you prepared for your very first baby steps when your proud parents gawked at you with anticipation day after day many years ago? If you could recall, you'd remember you were giggling, reaching and bouncing around with excited eyes like a lovable little nutso. Enthusiasm unbriddled by doubt was your only reference. Think as eagerly and positively about the year to come as you modestly add another to the numbers. Resistance is stressful and fatiguing. Ease into the active lifestyle, unbound and fearless, with that same bright smile and those innocent sparkling eyes. It can happen all over again, over time.

Do you have any hang-ups? Aren't they a drag? Should you dare fight convention and put order into your life, eat right and lift weights, they will grow faint, as surely as the early morning sun replaces the dark of night. It's true, almost poetic.

It's not uncommon in the world of the overweight for the dwellers to think unkindly of themselves, casting a reproving eye on their movements and the space they occupy. Get over it. This is your lot, the boundaries of your life, and here you will remain unless you befriend yourself, pardon yourself of past stumblings and refrain from inflicting further undeserved punishment. Twisted self-affliction damages the goods further, like taking a hammer to the toes of the feet that lost the race. The race is never lost as long as you continue to take another step forward.

I love this old world in spite of the violence, disease and politics. Take care of your own backyard and give your kind neighbor a hand when he needs it. Appreciate yourself with due humility for your strengths and be grateful, for as long as you apply your talent and integrity, you are making progress. Remember this, ye walking, talking, thinking and feeling miracle: Progress is not only measured in inches and pounds but also in what is not seen in external, physical structure. Don't fail to calculate the improved health of the internal system, i.e. the organs, hormones, enzymes and their interplay, and the subjective models of character in the mind—patience, determination and perseverance. A flood of improvement of far more value than the loss of a pound rushes on beneath the skin. Don't forget the delight of fulfillment and the thrill of success.

## The company you keep

Incidentally, if I'm not being too snoopy or snobby, with whom do you hang? An old friend of mine from Memphis wrote recently to make a point. Two years ago he and his wife moved to New Orleans, coincidentally just after she completed an arduous dieting program.

She had established a group of supportive friends and lost "130 pounds of you-know-what." He observes, "Talk about eating problems—barbecues in Memphis, Cajun cooking in New Orleans. Some of these people don't have a chance. They live to eat instead of eat to live. You really have to search to find a healthy food source. You have to search harder for people who give a darn."

He advises, "In order to overcome these obesity-related obstacles, you have to break away from the crowd. Birds of a feather flock together. You actually have to find new friends who don't have food on their mind 24/7. With her new job in New Orleans came new friends and no sign of diet consciousness. Beth gained the weight back in two years. Wrong companions, lost support and control. I have pictures to prove it."

I believe it. You can run, but you can't hide. You want to do this thing right? Get rid of your old family and friends, starting with your boss, then the spouse and after that…

Nah. Doesn't work that way, but awareness of the negative influences that surround you can help. You can prepare for the battle and fight it. Some days you win, and some you lose. That's life. Plop yourself down void of judgment and envy amid the good souls with whom you live, love, work and play. Observe their behavior with a quick eye and see yourself as one of them: a giddy participant, merrily eating and drinking for tomorrow you might die. Is this okay with you? I mean, they're good people and all, just living and socializing.

Good stands out like a light in the darkness. You're the strong one and might very well influence them. You're the star. Shine.

## Blood sugar swings

In simple terms the foods we eat are processed in the mouth, stomach and, eventually, the liver. Some nutrients are absorbed directly through the linings of the stomach and the intestines. For the most part they are hydrolyzed (broken down) in the liver into intrinsic elements (amino acids, glucose, vitamins, minerals, fiber and various metabolites) and transported throughout the body via the blood for their constructive work. Carbohydrate is converted into a simple sugar called glucose (a.k.a. blood sugar) where it is sent off to provide fuel for the brain and body. The glucose that is not burned directly as energy is stored as glycogen in the liver and muscle. Excessive intake of sugar is converted into fat. That's sort of the way it goes if everything is operating according to plan.

Maintaining a balance of sugar in our system is critical to our health. Imbalances contribute to sensitivity reactions—hyperactivity for example—to compound diseases such as diabetes. Low blood sugar (hypoglycemia) is a condition one might expect was reserved for the thin under-eater, yet it is often this condition common to overweight dieters that contributes to their obesity. The frustrated dieter often starves in an attempt to lose weight and thus suffers low-blood-sugar symptoms. The body reacts to the decrease of calories by slowing down the metabolism and storing energy as fat around the middle. What a revolting predicament this is.

How many struggling overweight folks eat without restraint (stuff themselves) over a carefree weekend and try to make up for it by starving themselves during the week? They become ill-tempered, impatient and run-down, wondering why they can't lose weight? And, if they do, they wonder why they're getting flabby, fatigued and building another chin. You see why, don't you? Of course. They lost prized muscle during the week and they stored burdensome fat over the weekend.

This is the notorious, downward spiral. Think about it, a frightening and oppressing conflict. Panic comes to my mind. Do you know anyone like this: a loved one, a spouse, a teammate or a child? Could it be you? This is a devastating sickness that needs to be fixed before it advances and it becomes too late. Can you talk to them? Will they listen? What can we do? The cure is sure, but takes action and courage. Ironically, it's free. Eat right and work out.

## Meet another pal

Say, have you met Liz? She's a star. Liz has been a member of our gym since we opened in 1989. After her baby boy was born, she was determined to lose the extra pounds she'd gained and certainly didn't want to become a "fat mom" as she called some of her girlfriends.

She casually but poignantly confided in me as we walked around the gym floor during her first visit, "Of me and my close friends, I'm the last to marry and have a baby. I've watched them change into busy, yet inactive, wives and moms, and they've lost something priceless in the transition. They either eat a lot or don't eat at all; they've lost daily structure and they've sort of given in to frustration. I don't think it's necessary."

She struggled to wring out an hour from her time-parched mothering schedule and confessed she was alone in her fight. "I love Tom. He's supportive, but works hard and he's not interested," she said, and her girlfriends were content as they continued to squeeze themselves into the plump social mold. She leaned close and whispered, as if someone might be eavesdropping, "I think they're lazy." The gym became her brief, daily refuge, and her desire to be strong and in shape became her expression. I praised her fortitude. We all did.

One day a bright, five-year-old guy, Butch, accompanied her to the gym "to see where Mommy lifts weights." Another guy about Liz's age tagged behind with his hands dug in his pockets. Tom was his name and he was Liz's knight in shining armor, her husband. I joined the party to share in the enthusiasm of my heroine (it was clear the dear girl needed help) and to demonstrate a few exercises to the men in her life. Tom was impressed and, after some secret family persuasion, he took the bar from the rack and performed his very first bench press. Liz and I moved on, and Butch helped his dad add some weights to the captivating bar. What a curious pair of playmates.

Liz and I looked at each other like we were stealing cherries as Tom later purchased a membership and made plans to work out the next morning. Tom now benches, squats and deadlifts regularly because, as he says, "There is nothing better than the basics." Two of Liz's girlfriends meet her during the week for the restoration of their bodies and minds. Everybody is getting in on the act. Butch sneaks in on the weekends.

## Get some help

How's your support system? I grew up when it was best if you didn't talk about your weird little pastime. "A muscle-bound waste of energy and time, boy." But, Coach. "You'll hurt yourself, son." Gee, Ma. I responded to the unconventional, and I thrived.

Today a support system is valuable—a challenging partner to share the workouts when the gym looks dreary or when it looks seriously exciting. Someone to keep you accountable and with whom to share your highs and lows, ask questions and discuss possibilities. I'm amazed at the abundance of real, honest and quality e-mail discussion groups there are on the Internet: inspiring, informed and intelligent. Some of these are listed in the resource appendix at the back of the book.

There are also personal trainers who can teach you, assist you and get you to the gym on time. Shop around 'cuz this is a budding career, and too many trainers are sweet, cute and toddling. Certificates they have. Understanding... maybe not. Look for experience through application, integrity and a special chemistry that engages. Be strong; leave the nest when you can fly.

The commercial group weight-loss programs give out a lot of information, guidance, pep talks, specific menus to follow, accountability processing and, sometimes, lists of foods to buy or in-house brands of foods to choose. Check these out carefully if you are convinced you can't do this alone. The message is basically the same: Eat right, exercise and stick to it. Join the crowd and do it together.

Eagles soar. I seldom see an eagle, never mind a flock.

Motivation must come from the heart. The brave act on the motivation. The long-suffering perform the hard work. The disciplined realize the reward. The humble give thanks.

## Junk and video games

*Innocent eyes peer from round faces*
*Too young to know the fight.*
*Soon smiles will be replaced by sad traces*
*Of a child against the obesity plight.*

*I should have known.*
*Why didn't they say?*
*How large you've grown;*
*I'd be strong today*

*I look at the vital world by my side.*
*It moves at a pace I cannot keep.*
*From healthy smiles I want to hide,*
*Between the cracks I wish to seep.*

*Continued...*

*There's hope for us, I heard someone say.*
*Exercise, eat right and start right away.*
*Please, record the refrain and push replay.*
*Exercise, eat right and start right away.*

Kids are forever. More than one-third of the nation's children are overweight and face chronic, debilitating health problems including heart disease, diabetes and cancer by their early 30s. They are scarred by insecurity and self-disappointment before they reach their teens. Life is a rocky road.

Studies done in California by the Berkeley-based Public Health Institute released findings in September 2000 that high schoolers are growing alarmingly fat and lazy on a diet of junk food and video games.

The researchers were disheartened by the statistics, pointing out, "This is the best time of their life; things are never going to get better than now and we really have to do something." The "something," of course, is very complicated. It involves legislation, bureaucracy, governments, schools, parents, kids, committees, persuasion, industry, greed, ignorance and stupidity.

The other thing, naturally, is diet and exercise.

Seventy percent of the rascals eat fast food like mom and dad, 30 percent don't eat fruit or vegetables (unless you call fries "veggies") and they also spend twice as much time watching television and playing video games as being physically active. School systems offer the ever-popular fast foods at their cafeterias, and physical education class attendence has dropped to disgraceful lows.

Something is terribly wrong with the societies around the world when we study the petri dish that is California. The scientists expected conditions to be considerably better in the "physical" California environment. A myth. They recommend a major public awareness campaign, and I'm all for that. How would that play out with the fast-food industry, however, and those conglomerates selling the junk? Not very well. Tobacco anyone?

The ball is rolling in the wrong direction, and those for whom weight-loss books are written need to get out of the way. The awareness is rising, yet the momentum of the ball is building. You must act on your own behalf and protect your children. Teach them through education, encouragement and, most of all, by your own behavior. Sweep the cupboards for them as well as for you. Set the table and eat together whenever you can. Hike, bike, take them to the gym, play and swim. Fight the fight in good cheer, never embarrassing, always promoting, bound for health, fitness and high spirits. Honest enthusiasm is contagious.

Like parent, like child. Bequeath them a sound and disciplined body.

## It's tuna and water time

I throw fastballs, curves and a mean change of pace, but you haven't seen my looptyloop. Get ready to duck.

The following technique is hardcore and doesn't follow the rules. Athletes—bodybuilders, in particular—practice this protein-exclusive principle to muscularize before competition. You are going to eat tuna and drink water for three straight days. Hissss… My, how quickly we lose our sense of humor.

You're cleaning house, fortifying the good habits and dismantling the bad. It's time to make a strong and definite statement before the audience that matters most. You. Take this short and tough departure for all it's worth: the test of will, a mind and body cleansing, the experience of a sudden and abrupt menu change that often initiates positive hormonal adjustment. More and more researchers are agreeing that sugar is the problem in the modern diet. Breaking the carb intake totally is good for you as you prepare for the unfolding long-term diet you're planning.

Goes like this: Choose your starting day. Psyche up. You'll be consuming water by the jugs—two to four liters a day—and one to one-and-a-half grams of protein per pound of body weight divided into six equal servings throughout the day. Back this with your vitamins and minerals two times a day, eight capsules of branch chain amino acids (key muscle-building protein) before and after your workouts, a gulp of EFA oil and a nightly portion of Metamucil for fiber.

Forget what you want, what you feel like and what you read. You are in the trenches on the front lines where you gain ground and make the difference. Your energy may dip before it rises, but your body chemistry will soon adapt. Be strong.

Incredible. We fret and agonize over our excessive body weight. We have for months or is it years? We gobble down all the fanciful diets offered by the most recent wave of experts or authorities. Asked to do the "Big One" and we fold. Well, almost. As needed grumble to yourself, but master your attitude. This harsh jumpstart never fails to kick in the metabolism and set the weight tumbling.

Later in the week bring in chicken, low-fat cottage cheese and salad or your favorite steamed vegetable to fortify your menu without expanding it significantly. You're feeding the muscle. Here's a delightful bedtime snack: tuna from the can, scoop of cottage cheese and cool, clear water. Combine this with some naturally released growth hormone during your deep sleep and presto.

Live life and exercise lightly to accommodate a temporary low-calorie strength loss. Press on as the body adapts and as you become familiar and confident. This is a rigid practice to test your resolve, investigate your chemistry, break some troublesome habits and narrow ever-widening margins. It will bring you to the doorstep of the ketogenic diet where protein intake, exclusive of carbs, creates a ketone-burning system for energy.

Extreme measures…

# Chapter 14

## Special Reports:
### Diabetes, Heart Disease, Cancer & the Fast-Food Industry

Some things, as ordinary as they seem, are worth repeating. We are all different, and we all have different reasons for wanting to lose weight. Whatever they are today, the day will come in each our lives when we realize that none are more important than health and long life. If a trimmer body, abdominal muscles, a two-piece or size six aren't enough motivation to rid yourself of fat and fattening ways, perhaps you'll find the purpose in these brief reports—life itself, precious, full of wonder and fleeting. Listen to the dark and ominous tones of ignorance, irresponsibility and neglect. Shame is not my intention, and I don't care to heap guilt on anyone. I want you to right what's wrong and fix what's broken before it's too late. Act now. The clock is ticking.

I have listed the top four maladies associated with obesity. One is as grim as the other and one appears to be on the wrong list. Well, not exactly.

## Diabetes

Let's begin with diabetes as it is the most recent monster to claim control of the overweight societies across the planet. In America 16 million people suffer from diabetes, a 40-percent rise in the past decade. Nearly all have a form of the disease called Type 2 diabetes that's largely associated with obesity and inactivity.

The disease is complex, and the research tackling the problem is vast. A large portion of the food we eat is converted into glucose, or sugar, for our energy needs. Insulin, a hormone produced in the pancreas, assists glucose into the cells where its energy goes to work. When a person is diabetic, either the pancreas doesn't make enough insulin for healthy glucose transportation or the cells begin to resist insulin. Fat is the core of insulin resistance and actively produces resistin, an energy-conserving hormone, which interferes with insulin's task to carry sugar into the cells. Hence, the cells don't get enough energy, and worse, glucose and insulin build up in the blood vessels and damage the arterial walls. Circulation is impaired, and a long list of trouble begins.

The American Diabetes Association points out, "People with diabetes have a four-fold increase of cardiovascular events like heart attacks and strokes. Diabetes causes nerve damage throughout the body, making it the leading cause of blindness, lower-extremity amputations and end-stage renal failure."

Diabetes is epidemic, as is obesity. This disabling disease is directly related to society's overweight condition and its inactivity. The message is loud and clear to the diabetes community. Lose weight. Exercise, eat right and smile. Do it for good.

We are quick to squirm and pass the buck to our Mom and Pop and their Mom and Pop, the ever popular "gene routine." Try this on for size: Behavior largely determines your health—what you eat, what you do, today and tomorrow and forever. More often than not, you can fix what's broken, strengthen it or prevent it from breaking. It's up to you.

Exercise ultimately increases the body's ability to absorb sugar, and eating right means less sugar consumption and less overeating at a single sitting. The two together provide promise for a less-fat, more-muscled body with an improved metabolism and systemic chemistry. Imagine, a loss of as little as 5-percent body weight by eliminating sugar alone can turn around a suffering diabetic.

The National Institute of Health is involved in the cure of diabetes and the Center for Disease Control focuses on informing the public of diseases and assuring that countermeasures are put into daily practice. Ironically, the concern is whether the people waste the information gained by the research and study? When it comes to lifestyle and behavioral changes, will the threatened creature choose the path to years of good health or ignore the life-saving recommendations and stumble along like a fool. The apathy of modern, settled societies is absolutely scary.

One third of the 16 million diabetics in the United States don't realize they have the disease. A straightforward blood test reveals the truth, but few people take it. The symptoms listed by the International Sports Sciences Association include frequent urination, excessive thirst, unexplained changes in weight, frequent hunger, sudden vision changes, tingling or numbness in hands and feet and chronic fatigue. Sometimes nausea and stomach pains occur. Sound familiar? See your doctor.

Ten years ago diabetes seldom afflicted the youth. Today, one out of 50 kids has Type 2 diabetes; the number is rising, and the age range is down to three and four-year-olds. Obesity is the underlying problem, and the culprit is the behavior that brought about the fatness: junk food in the mouth and TV in the face. The kids don't have a chance if the parents and role models don't rise up and run the race. You don't have to win or be in the top 10; just get up and run. The kids will tag along. They love to tag along. Thirty years from now we'll be on our knees if we don't get moving.

## Heart disease

Responding to a newsletter I sent to IronOnline.com subscribers outlining the *Your Body Revival* book project, a reader remarked that reaching the overweight crowd was a futile cause. "They are lost to bad habits, weakened will and denial," she claimed. One reader asked a good question: "Who will buy the book?" Another applauded my concern with a speck of condescension and doubt, as if I, being spiritial and all, had suddenly witnessed unmuscled, oversized people and thought they needed saving. Huh?

Bulletin. I'm going on a hundred years old and 20 years into recovering from severe congestive heart failure—seems the old boy drank too much Moonshine for a spell. The Bomber, a pillar of clay, needed re-girding and the lessons in reconstruction are mighty and unforgettable. How do they go again? You reap what you sow. Garbage in, garbage out. You are responsible for your body; respect it. Denial destroys. Procrastination paralyzes.

Heart attack, stroke and other diseases of the heart are now among the leading causes of death. The secret's been out for a century and, though heart disease can be traced in our genes, much of it is by our own hand. Again the research and statistics and cost in human suffering are staggering. And it rises. Are we incorrigible?

I feel like a pest. No one wants to be badgered. It certainly is easier to dismiss the subject and talk about sports, the job, your favorite sitcoms and recipes. Allow me a few tiny reminders, okay? Any cigarettes at all, a little too much alcohol, way too much fat and sugar, and far too little activity contribute to our tragedy. Arteries that move our blood are closing down, circulation is insufficient for menial activity and we're only 35, going on 40. You haven't begun to live and can't run across the street to avoid oncoming traffic. The low-density lipoprotein (LDL, the "bad" cholesterol) is up and the high-density lipoprotein (HDL, the "good" cholesterol) is down. The weight is up and the exercise is down. Anxiety is up and contentment is down. Blood pressure is up, composure down. Carelessness is up and caring for yourself is down. Do not follow the masses over the edge.

## Cancer

Cancer research marches on and slowly the onionskins are peeled away. As in the study of the solar systems, the more space we cover the more distant and numerous the objects of wonder revealed. The research is vast. We're learning, but it takes so long to link the minds and determine the cross-section of goals; decide methods of operation; run long-term studies with impossible variables; and staff, fund, govern, record and evaluate. How does it get done?

What do I know about cancer? Enough to know that it kills suddenly or slowly and whomever it pleases. None of us is immune; we are all at risk, and we who throw up a shield to its randomly swinging sword are valiant warriors. Our scientist friends assure us that living a healthy lifestyle—curiously the same as the one I praise in these straight-talking pages—gives us a significantly better chance at out-maneuvering the grim opponent.

We are at more risk across the board for a list of cancers when obesity clutches our life. It is not the condition itself, but the sorry foods consumed achieving obesity that account for cancers, including endometrial cancer, breast cancer, cancer of the colon and gastrointestinal cancers. Though research has not been sufficient to prove that obesity increases the risk of cancer or weight loss reduces the risk of cancer, studies in late 2001 by the World Health Organization have the doctors of the panel suitably convinced obesity plays a significant role in the plight. Indiscriminate diets high in saturated fat, high in sugar and low in fiber are associated with an increased the risk of cancer.

There is speculation that exercise and high-fiber diets contribute to the efficient passage of waste products through the digestive tract, giving carcinogens less time to act upon the lining of the colon.

Estrogen is produced in fat cells, and the greater the volume of body fat, the more estrogen present in a woman's system. It is believed that the greater the exposure to estrogen, the greater the woman's risk of breast cancer.

It's obvious. I'm not invested in the knowledge in this field to speak with intelligence—I daresay there is a lot of hypothesis and educated guessing when dealing in the dark—but haven't you noticed that our treatment of this phenomenon, the human body, is unpardonably sloppy? We are more attentive and particular in the care of our poodle.

Someone once speculated that were we paid by the hour to care properly for ourselves we would surely do a better job. But offer us life itself in payment and we hesitate.

## The fast-food industry

How did I know 40 years ago that "fast food," the vulgar, insidious preparation of chicken, beef, fish and potatoes with its accompanying slurpy beverages, was bad for me? I felt the same way about slippery green snakes that hissed in the grass. It was something in the way they wiggled, shimmered and shined.

The inception of the fast-food restaurant goes back 50 years and its history and evolution is fascinating. You can read sanitized chronicles of the young entrepreneurs who rose from struggling immigrant backgrounds, poor farm families and the ranks of high school dropouts to start Carl's Jr., Wendy's, Kentucky Fried Chicken, Burger King and the big daddy, McDonald's. The vision, determination and persistence they shared is remarkable; their competitive nature singular. Remove the bun, the lettuce, tomato and secret sauce and you see the real meat of the story.

The American free market spawned the hamburger joints that delighted the palates of the common man, suited his pocket and coincided with his need for convenience and life on the go. The fast-food restaurants, more like pit stops, took off one after another, grew side by side and soon piled on top of each other. The race was on, and the numbers of participants swamped the field.

What happened to barbecues in the backyard and dinner at home with the family?

Fast food has covered the planet like moss and challenged mankind's health. It's put a chink in the armor of the vanishing individual and propagated the grinning, baying masses. The profile of the economy has been rearranged by the powerful industry and its many and long-reaching tentacles. Where there is immense power and growth, so is there politics and favors, oversight and corruption.

The top players will do anything to expand their businesses—to one another, to you and me. I'm wagging my finger at all of us as we come from the same human pool; we sit on opposite sides of the seesaw, but together we keep the super-fat machine in motion. They produce; we consume. Which came first: the McChicken or the McEgg?

Let's take a quick look:

All the food in a fast-food restaurant is frozen, dehydrated, condensed, highly processed and freeze dried. It is full of fat, sugar, salt and preservatives. Secret flavors prepared in laboratories account for the taste appeal of the fries, meat and milkshakes. Without them you would doubt their authenticity as food. A mouth-watering strawberry shake at Burger King contains 48 different chemicals with names like benzyl isobutyrate and ethyl methlphenylglycidate. I'll have wa-ter and a napkin; please, hold the food.

The fast-food industry loves the government as long as it can govern it, usurp it or dodge it. It gets considerable tax breaks for hiring unskilled workers whom it promises to train and doesn't. It underpasy its teen workforce, does nothing to develop them as "Young America," loses them before insurance and vacation benefits accrue and gener-ally uses them up. Okay, what's the point? It's not right, and I thought you might be interested.

How about this? Fast food is in school cafeterias with all its un-balanced and nocuous ingredients. Just what little Tommy and Susie need to grow fat, hypered and insulin-dependent. It's also perfect tim-ing to develop their taste for fat and syrup to ensure that they reach for the junk the rest of their lives. Who let this stuff in the schools in the first place?

We swing into the wide parking lot beneath the golden arches, gang in tow and make our order of jumbo Cokes (310 calories), super-size fries (610 calories—29 grams of fat) and double burgers with cheese and bacon (about 1,000 calories—45 grams of fat). The kids are off in the red, yellow and blue plastic playground, sliding down slopes and planning the toys they'll snag on the way out the door. One hundred million McHappy Meals were sold in 10 days during a record-break-ing Teenie Beanie Baby giveaway. Thanks, Mom, do I get to keep all the fat and calories, too? How about the degenerating habits?

Yes, I know, you're right. Sociology is neither my expertise nor the scope of this book, but I'm learning. The relevance of man's greed, power and ego, along with his ignorance and denial, cannot be ex-cused from the unresolved condition he faces today: unchecked, self-destructive, weak-willed obesity. It's been thrust upon us by our-selves. I simply want you to know the source of some of the problems. Understanding a problem can help with its solution.

I hope my plea, statements and non-revolutionary solutions make it outside the borders of my home, but I will reference America, as the Stars and Stripes seems to be leading in the problems I address. Fur-thermore, the research here is available. The United States has the highest rate of obesity in the world—about 40 million adults are obese, a 60-percent increase in just the last 10 years. About 20 percent of the population is over 30 pounds in the red zone and one third of our kids are overweight and out of shape. There are an alarming seven million folks walking around who are ranked as super obese and weigh at least a hundred pounds more than normal. A fat and unfit nation has locked hands with the fast-food culture, a death grip that needs to be loosened.

There is no definitive epidemiological study that proves the relationship between obesity and the fast-food restaurants. I'm just haunted by this nagging suspicion and the coincidence. Fast-food restaurants spread like wildfire in the late '60s and early '70s with the obesity epidemic trailing in its billowing haze. McDonald's leaped the seas and opened shop in Great Britain, doubling its outlets throughout the years of 1985 to 1995. It was noted that the obesity rate of our great ally doubled as well.

Japan and China have not been spared. These once lean and healthy nations are growing pouches wholesale. Century upon century, these rigorous and crowded populations have not indulged in the excesses of the material life. There are a multitude of benefits from too little or just enough—starvation keeps mankind lean, and prevents and kills many diseases.

Modernized and less repressed, the people are eating freely and need to be on the alert for diseases they've never before known: heart disease, stroke, diabetes...you know the list. They also need to be on the alert to eat right and prevent the development of bad (modern) eating habits.

Obesity is hard to cure, and some researchers believe prevention is the best remedy. I believe it is part of the prescription, but it will not fix what's broken today as we desperately seek a healthier, more agreeable weight. Resisting a brightly lit, aroma-filled Jack in the Box serving fat, sugar and chemicals in abundance is a good practice. Hurry. A new fast-food restaurant opens every two hours.

# Fast Food Nation

The economy is supporting the fast-food trend and fast food has become a major industry. Fifty billion dollars a year are spent on advertising the slop. The government of the United States spends one flea-sized million to remind us that we need to eat more fruit and vegetables. It's a crying shame: A few billion tax dollars fall through some bureaucratic cracks while we desperately need nationwide education.

Incidentally, another 20 billion a year is spent on candy ads. If you sniff around, something smells and it isn't home cooking.

If you want to read a cool book tracking the fast-food industry and disclosing its global affects, pick up a copy of *Fast Food Nation* by Eric Schlosser. Extensively researched by the award-winning journalist, the pages move along and are written with heart.

# Chapter 15

## Hormones Everywhere:
### *The Governing System*

Plowing over stacks of research like a stubborn workhorse, rummaging through my muscle-building memory and scratching out a scheme to help you lose fat is not an easy task. I accept the mission gratefully. It is worth every bit of my time, energy and sacrifice to be in any way a part of your success. However, the information, facts, biochemistry, sequences of hormonal and enzyme activity, and the interrelationship of nutrients in the bodies of healthy and unhealthy men and women, though pertinent and logical, are confusing when presented in a small book intending to be direct, charged and inspirational. Difficulty also arises when the reader is not a pre-med student but simply a guy or gal interested in losing some undesired fat and screaming for help.

The time has come for me to lay out in blasphemous simplicity the importance of the body's key hormones and their role in energy, fat storage, muscle building and disease. I must present it with originality and clarity, fact and conviction if you are to read and believe what I say. Okay, here goes: Once upon a time long, long ago, there lived a happy, thriving family of hormones in the magical body of a jolly ole fat man. On a bright and sunny morning when he bent over to put on his shoes, he discovered he couldn't reach his feet. "Oh, my," he said, "What am I going to do?" Little did he know that...

Hormones, vast in number and comprising an intricately connected system, are considered by scientists to be the body's most powerful biological agents, regulating almost entirely the chemical activities of the body. Their handiwork is reflected in the storage and distribution of excess body fat, the density and strength of muscle, levels of energy and sex drive, and the symptoms of aging. The foods we ingest are immediately attended by these amazing workers, and they can serve us both positively and negatively. We can, at some point and to a large degree, control the activity of the hormones to optimize their affects on our health and longevity.

The five hormones on which I have selected to sketch a rough profile are growth hormone, testosterone, insulin, glucagon and cortisol.

**Growth hormone**, produced in the pituitary gland, is particularly involved in building muscle and directing the body to burn fat. Keep in mind that any efficiency we have in building, repairing and replacing muscle is also efficiency in retarding the aging process. Growth hormone cooperates well with insulin and testosterone in building muscle. This life-giving ingredient enhances immune function and inhibits early stages of arteriosclerosis along with numerous symptoms of aging. Growth hormone is secreted in the early hours of deep sleep and during specific periods of intense exercise; it unfortunately declines in production as one gets older.

**Testosterone** is the super hormone in man responsible for his sexuality and male characteristics. It is, to a much lesser degree, present in women. It plays a powerful role in muscle building and fat burning and, like growth hormone, production declines with age. Testosterone levels fluctuate and can be increased by exercise, providing overtraining is not initiated and environmental variables (fitness, nutrition and eating patterns, rest, sleep and emotional stress) are favorably controlled.

**Insulin** is the hormone secreted by the pancreas. Its principal purpose is to transport blood sugar into the cells for energy. It also moves amino acids into the tissues for their anabolic action. Not incidentally, insulin in excess is a very potent fat-storage agent, a fat builder. Any given person is more or less insulin resistant or insulin sensitive, depending on a wide variety of conditions including obesity, lack of exercise, excessive sugar intake, insufficient dietary fat, emotional stress and genetic predisposition.

Insulin resistance is fast becoming the medical problem of this day and age. When carbohydrates are eaten excessively, insulin remains chronically high and the cells eventually adapt to its presence and become resistant to its function; additional insulin is demanded to continue its job. The persistent and long-term elevation of insulin and glucose in the bloodstream causes havoc in the system. We want insulin in our system only when we need it, not because we glut ourselves with sugary foods. It should be noted that insulin and growth hormone are mutually antagonistic. We want growth hormone in our system whenever it knocks on our door, not to be turned away by the intrusive presence of insulin.

**Glucagon** is also a secretion of the pancreas, yet it is exactly opposite of insulin in its action. Glucagon converts glycogen to blood sugar, whereas insulin converts blood sugar to glycogen. Glycogen is unused glucose stored in either muscle tissue or the liver to serve as energy when needed. Low blood sugar signals glucagon production, stimulating glycogen conversion to glucose to be transported to the cells by insulin. Should insulin resistance, engendered by over-consumption in general and of sugar in particular, interfere with the cells' uptake of glucose, we have a perfect setup for obesity and Type 2 diabetes, with lots of sugar and ineffective insulin in the blood.

To simplify, if you followed the order of events of macronutrient ingestion to their active place in the bloodstream, you would find that, eventually, excess insulin stores fat and glucagon mobilizes or burns fat. This can be a positive and healthy process if care in the initial manner, quality and quantity of ingestion is observed. Careless eaters risk chaotic blood sugar levels, appetite cravings, adipose development and loss of muscle. Mood swings and energy dips often accompany over-consumption and misguided blood sugar reservoirs.

**Cortisol:** Where growth hormone and testosterone are hormones that promote muscle building, life extension, well-being, immunity, resistance, energy and fat burning, cortisol is the catabolic hormone that destroys muscle and contributes to undesirable fat storage. It is primarily a product of stress, both real and imaginary. Stress prompts its release from the adrenal cortex and floods our system 24/7. Over-training elevates cortisol levels; lack of sound sleep facilitates its destructive action, and we find it everywhere at once competing with and compromising testosterone and growth hormone anabolic action. Nutrition, sleep, stress-buffering attitude and exercise counter the enemy.

Behold the battle. Complex and fascinating or just confusing, the undeniable fact is that hormones rule. Piece the puzzle together hormone by hormone or look at the picture on the box; the impression is the same. Exercise, eat right for good and the hormones will probably fall in their proper place. The underlining recommendation to assist healthy hormonal function is to get in shape and stay the course—another miracle of science and common sense.

You have just read my distillation of the raw material available to us in volumes of medical research dedicated to the metamorphosis of man and to his diseased or healthy condition. Those hormones are a busy bunch. I offer the last dozen painful paragraphs for you to ponder, hold in your mental shirt pockets and reference from time to time as telltale words pop up in muscle talk and beg explanation. My synopsis of the underlying activities of fat storage, muscle growth and hormones might shed some light in the dark corners where secrets are hidden. Or not. (I slept at a Holiday Inn Express last night.)

## The secrets lurk in dark dungeons

Preparing a book of instruction based on research, documentation, experience and musing is an unfolding process. That is, you learn new facts, recall ground once covered and arrive at new conclusions, as well as gain reassurance about original ideas. Occasionally, amid the compiling of information, an insight penetrates you like a flash. Remember the first time you accidentally whistled or really noticed the difference between a boy and a girl? Well, something like that.

Let me recount something I noticed while reviewing my early training and diet experimentation. In the early '60s, there were few solid facts to follow, and one relied on trial and error to set one's course—arguably more direct and less confusing than today where stacks of sophisticated information abound. Unlike you, I was confronted with the difficult process of gaining body weight that begged for muscular size and shape. At 6-feet and 230 pounds, I was seeking to gain another 20 pounds of bulk.

I know; you should have such a problem. Hang on for a second, as I have a story to tell and a point to make that validates the menu and diet plan I advocate for you. I believe it will help you understand.

The year was 1963. I was a recent New Jersey transplant in Santa Monica, California, where the remnants of Muscle Beach resided. The beach scene had receded, but the bodybuilding energy, learning and growing had not. The atom was accelerating. I, by osmosis, took on the training principles that dominated the iron game during this shift from the beach to the Dungeon, the new underground digs for the relocated muscleheads. (Seems the city council didn't understand their behavior.) Powerlifting was infiltrating the ranks of the slick bodybuilders and super-size was gaining popularity. At the same time, none of us wanted to sacrifice muscle definition; at least, we wanted to retain as much as we could while packing on the pounds. Some things never change.

This was accomplished according to one's own madness, although there were common threads that weaved through the menus of the progressive lifters—high protein and low carbs with the fats relatively high in that red meat, eggs and milk products were primary ingredients. Salads were big-time favorites and tuna fish somehow took on an importance similar to that of oxygen. The bad boys carried jugs of water. There were no girls, by the way.

Notice the trend being set by the greatest researchers this side of the moon. Protein: high. Fat: medium. Carbs: low.

I set off to gain weight and get strong while expecting the muscular size to grow according to the big food intake and the intense, power-accented, bodybuilding regimens. It worked. It took time, hard work, patience, discipline and perseverance. These, too, I accumulated along the way. It was during my recent recollections that I recognized a component of the mass-seeking process that coincidentally matched recent scientific consensus.

Bulking up day in and day out can be as difficult as dieting down. It can be as frustrating and delirious, as disheartening and dull. I eventually, through survival and need of relief, began a practice of eating with stoic deliberation during the week to serve me and power me through my work and workouts. The hard-core bulking phase came on the weekends when time and relaxation were to be found and smorgasbord specials were in abundance at the best coastal restaurants. I packed in the calories in all shapes and sizes on Saturday and Sunday. I ate very well, until my eyes bulged.

There were additional attributes beyond the variety and change of pace: I was exceedingly strong for several days after the bulking phase and capitalized on this in the gym for big and heavy workouts; I was tight and pumped with great satisfaction and had a sense of overall well-being. I did this regularly for three years. Two to three months out of the year when the summer rolled around and competition or photo sessions were in the works, the muscle-defining techniques were implemented. I deduced that the added weight included a percentage of muscle mass accounting for the increased power, energy and well-being; the pump came from the fuel provided by the carbs; and the tightness came from the bloat of body weight. The logic, which I shared with my buddies, was reasonably correct on all accounts.

We're getting close to my pea-brain observation.

The popular diets that interest me today as I see them laid out in books and booklets are the ones that endorse this system of steady, healthy food intake in the balances I instinctively prefer (high protein, plenty of mixed fats and relatively low carbohydrate) for five days followed by a heavy loading phase for one or two days; anything goes. Sound familiar?

The proponents of these diet procedures are doctors, researchers and recognized experts in the muscle-building and nutritional fields. These men and women go further than I in explaining the facts behind the muscle-building, fat-burning properties of this up-down feeding mechanism. It has been discovered that the hormones intricately involved in muscular growth—testosterone, growth hormone and insulin—are positively impacted by the scheme. That's the central point. These body-shaping and energy-producing hormones can be manipulated by your eating plan to bring about the changes you seek. The fix to your overweight dilemma goes beyond losing weight by dropping your calorie intake and walking the dog. The hormones hold the key.

What I perceived as bulking up for two days until I was satisfied (actually, I couldn't stand the discomfort and bloat any longer) turns out to have been an undeveloped and unheralded version of the famous hormone-adjusting, muscle-building plans put forth by Dr. Fred S. Hatfield, developer of the Zigzag Diet, and Dr. Mauro Di Pasquale, author of *The Metabolic Diet;* and comprehensively explained by genius Rob Faigin, author of *Natural Hormonal Enhancement.*

As scientifically suggested by the wise and studious educators, the bulking phase brings in a surge of carbs, stimulates insulin production, and causes cellular hydration and intracellular carbohydrate loading. This is an ideal environment of intense anabolic stimulus, yet it has a short efficiency span that needs to be determined experimentally by each of us.

How does the bulk up phase that I practiced 40 years ago apply to you, whose heart's desire is to lose weight... you, who have difficulty uttering the horrible expression "bulk up"? Briefly, without referring to the term one more time, I shall ellucidate: Establish your calorie intake to meet your minimum daily requirement: That is, your body weight times 12 to 15 calories. This is an approximation to guide you only. The important rule is that you follow the *Standard Balanced Menu* (see page 91-92) in your food arrangement to ensure you of those macronutrient balances that will positively affect your hormonal health.

Once you are comfortably practicing the trimmed and treated menu, begin to lower the caloric intake by 300-500 calories per day. This modification, along with moderate resistance exercise, provides the formula for weight loss, muscle stimulation and health improvement, including balanced hormonal chemistry.

Stable in diet and sound of mind, prepared for risk and in need of a good stretch, eat as you please over the weekend, no holds barred (I can't help it. I feel like I'm letting you play in traffic. Put a cap of, say, 2,000 extra calories per day on the madness, please... no, make that 1,000...use your judgment. I can't look.) and resume your weekday, calorie-rigid plan on Monday. The two days of relaxed eating and influx of carbohydrate stimulates the hormones (including insulin, glucagon and growth hormone) into an optimal fat-burning, muscle-building posture. Remember? Sugar-charged muscle cells pro-mote a training advantage for several uplifted days engendering the positive hormonal presence of growth hormone and testosterone. This bristling of the hormones under the perceived stress of macronutrient overload, likewise, arouses favorable hormone action.

The outline of my current menu is on page 82 in the chapter on boring menus. It's a good one; I like it and obviously recommend some version of it for you. The high-protein, medium-fat and rela-tively low-carb diet is the most sensible working diet for an overweight person who complements his life with muscle and strength-building exercise. Underlining the precept, "We are all different," you need to modify the scheme to suit yourself. That is done by simple trial and error and feel. You remain in control where you belong. I hope by now you do not wish to remain in the hands of a stranger.

It is here that you might bend a page to reference later as stuff continues to fall into place. Be it sufficient that you equip yourself with the elementary tools emphasized in the very next chapter. They are the stars that rule the universe of health, shape and might. The benefits of the zigzag diet pattern can be revisited just in time to resurge your interest and add a pleasing curve to the straight line.

## Apparent contradictions

I offer several ways to achieve weight loss, each of which is sub-ject to the exercise-and-eat-right principle. One way is to apply discipline in eating and training without interruption, being patient and hopeful that the discipline will grow and the fat will diminish over time. Little or no deviation from your rigid diet and training scheme is a built-in safeguard preventing you from wandering in ever-widening circles. This is tough, hardcore dieting; the standard that works, but makes few friends.

Some of you need choices and options and wider margins in your eating scheme or the terrain beneath your feet becomes unstable and impassable; misery in travel steers you to more comfortable ground, the slippery downward paths of no return. Beware.

Another method, riskier and more intricate, is to diet hard (a sufficient and wisely balanced diet) during the week and boost your food intake over the weekend. This boost offers relief to the struggling dieter and increases the ingredients that provide an anabolic or muscle-building environment in the body. A thoughtful increase of carbohydrates and protein positively affect the hormonal system ensuring hardy exercise and muscle growth through the days of the week that follow. The nature of this hormone-enhancing technique requires that muscle building and exercise are an established part of your weight-loss goal.

The extremes I offer appear to contradict each other. They are, in fact, different routes to similar destinations that I have practiced in the past and still do today, according to my needs, urges and desired affects. They are not exclusive of each other; that is, they can be alternated or blended to bring about desired fat-loss affects, each acting as a check or balance to prevent excessive eating, excessive dieting or exercise burnout. Complicated? No more than driving a stick shift. You'll get the hang of it. A most reliable vehicle to get you there. Automatics get stuck in the mud.

**This may be just the combination of order
and freedom you require and desire.**

# Surf's up, pump's up, weight's down

The day he joined the gym Lee weighed 250 at 5'4" and could move a house. In fact, to be precise, he planned and built houses in the valleys of central California when he wasn't riding big waves. Getting up on a surfboard became increasingly difficult and carrying his nail bags across scaffolding was downright dangerous. Changes had to be made: "I was a few months away from using a barge for a surfboard," he was heard to say.

Karaoke, anyone? Lip-sync the line while I play the tape. "Work out, eat right and carry on." Lee rearranged his eating habits and dropped his food intake from 4,500 greasy and sugary calories to 3,500 attractive, well-shaped units of energy. He did this with the patience and conscientiousness that accompanies carpenters, surfers and large children—till he got bored. It's okay, he thought, because he lost 30 pounds of beans and beer in six months.

I can see fading enthusiasm and wandering focus a mile away and a day early. Another month or two—through the winter and heading toward spring—he'd be hooked for good, I could tell. However, Lee's days of working out and eating right were numbered unless I grabbed him by the ears and hollered, which I did. "You quit now and I'll take a bite out of your long board. I'll hide your hammer and bend nails." You've gotta go for the jugular.

He grinned as I laid out my plan. "Everybody gets stale, we all lose interest and change might be the solution," I explained. "A short, planned layoff can be wise, but if you start carelessly missing your workouts, Lee, you'll sink. Let's talk." And we did, discussing his menu, training and some logical ebb-and-flow modifications. Lee's menu reasonably mimicked the Standard Balanced Menu (smart guy for a surfer). Fine. His calories hung at 3,500 regularly, down from his former ill-gotten 4,500 of the recent summer.

The plan staggered Lee's caloric intake to alter his even pace and flat playing field. Order is essential, and routine amid confusion is life preserving, but sameness suffocates. The caloric consumption remained the same during the first workweek (3,500) but was raised a brazen thousand calories (4,500) on the weekends with Lee eating carbs liberally to free his soul and load his glycogen stockpile. Monday morning of the second workweek he lowered his daily calorie intake by a hundred to a simmering 3,400 (mild caloric deficit) and maintained that number through the week. Monday and Tuesday his strength and energy soared due to the upload of resources, and the muscles brilliantly responded. He took advantage of the windfall and trained correspondingly. During the latter part of the week his training matched the natural dip in his endurance, complements of the daily 100-calorie reduction, as a pleasant fatigue set in. He lowered the weight he used and did thoughtful reps, his pre-workout meal faithfully carrying him along the way.

He repeated the weekend splurge with a grin and entered the new week with another 100-calorie drop (now 3,300). The weekend feasting afforded the all-time great workouts, and then Lee started to adjust to the weekday calorie decreases. The practice went on till 3,000 calories marked a sensible and comfortable number to balance regularly. He continued with renewed enthusiasm as he acknowledged his persistence in the face of submission. By mid-summer he was under 210 and felt like an oak. Dieting was no longer "dieting" after his ninth month of riding the iron waves. It was a solid and reassuring habit. Exercise became as familiar as his tools and surfboard, and easily as important.

Lee trains with the understanding and instinct that lives in all of us as we barrel forward to accomplish the tough things ahead of us. He manages his diet and exercise to accommodate his life. Thirty-seven years old with a family he started at 20, he consistently rolls along. All together now, "Eat right, train hard, be happy."

# Chapter 16

## Summarizing My Nutritional Plan:
### *Getting the Ducks in Order*

Time to conclude my presentation on nutrition, diet, menus and associated matters. I've told you what I've seen, read and done and what works for me and those around me. And I've underscored what doesn't work. You might be scratching your head, mouth ajar, because I didn't lay out in exact order what you should do. Well, that's not fair and, so, I affix a few signposts and emphasize the distinct landmarks in the summary below.

I'm hoping that in pointing you in the right direction, I'm helping you to cut your own path. That's the only honest, practical and comfortable way to reach your goal. Exactness is for technicians; it's wearisome and stifles the creative spirit. Pursuit of a healthy weight, a strong body and a good life is continual. Adding to your years and subtracting from your plight is instinctive.

**1.** Be ready for lifestyle changes. If that scares you, think it over. Take your time, and adopt changes gradually. What are the consequences if you don't?

**2.** Those changes are to include exercise. My input on that feature of the plan is coming up shortly. I know… you've got the chills.

**3.** Make some tangible evaluation of your physical condition. At least the bathroom scale and a sense of your mass, strength and well-being. You need to make reference points for future observation.

**4.** Make a list of your average daily food intake. By your choice you must:

- Eat breakfast, however small.

- Begin to serve yourself smaller meals more frequently.

- Avoid long periods (more than four hours) without eating.

- Begin to trim down portion sizes.

- Lower the carbohydrate and simple sugar intake.

- Increase your protein intake.

- Avoid excessive saturated fat (skin on chicken, fat in meat).

- Avoid deep-fried foods.

- Supplement your diet with a high quality vitamin and mineral and antioxidant formula.

- Include essential fatty acids (EFAs).

- Limit alcohol intake.

- Increase consumption of water to two quarts daily.

- Limit salt intake.

**5.** Care for yourself by being productive and active daily to stifle stress and promote well-being. Productive activity is fulfilling, heightens metabolism and calms the mind.

**6.** Get plenty of rest.

**7.** Vividly and positively imagine your goals and progress.

I've alluded to the alterations you can effect with your diet. The application of these practices puts those changes in motion. Ridding yourself of the sugar, providing strong inputs of protein and eating controlled portions regularly are the major players. Time and the investment of the aforementioned habits are the playing field. You're the MVP. Exercise is the name of the game. Let's play.

# Chapter 17

## Exercise Straight Talk:
### *Welcome to Revitalizing Exercise*

This and the next few chapters deal with the fascinating subject of exercise, one of the absolutes in the simple equation to solve the overweight problem.

Through the '60s physical education was required and taught in all schools. Today only half the schools offer it. Sports are passively watched and hardly played except by a few local leagues, the cream of high schools and colleges and, of course, the almighty pros. Once out of school the number of regular sports participants and exercise buffs drops to about zero, along with the level of fitness.

This is a relatively recent phenomenon and a great upheaval to the balance and health of mankind. You know the sad story. We are all part of it as we notice the electronic conveniences, high-tech mechanisms and video distractions taking charge of our lives. I beleaguer the point in hopes to strike a chord.

Qs...Are you excited that we "straight talkers" are finally on the verge of weight training and muscle building? Is your heart beating like a little kid's the night before Christmas at the thought of aggressively attacking the body fat with gym equipment in your hands? Or are you unconvinced that permanent weight loss is dependent upon building muscle mass, and are you intent upon proving me wrong?

As...I suspect many of you are former lifters getting back to the weights after a layoff of years and you yearn for that old-time feeling. Boomers, no doubt, comprise another large percentage of *Your Body*

*Revival* readers who grew up knowing of "The Blond Bomber" (me) as a bodybuilding nutso in the muscle mags of the '60s. You still lift on and off, have renewed your love for life and want to care for it a long, long time. You need to get back to the roots.

Here's a possibility: You're 30-something, never been in a gym, have been overweight all your life and enough is enough. I visualize men and women who are perhaps 50 pounds overweight and who want to fix what they can by taking some tough and determined steps because they're tough and determined. I only hope the teens who need to lose weight are also on the other side of this page and taking the steps for good to save themselves from the unnecessary struggle. Hard work is civilized. Hard work is cool.

You're in the midst of reading what I have to offer; assimilating the suggestions and proposals, rehashed facts and figures; wading through the threats and consequences: groping for some motivation or an accidental secret. Hold on for a minute and review the goals you outlined early on. Have they grown in substance? Are they still realistic or do they need revision? I don't want you to set yourself up for disappointment. I mean to push you and drag you but not shove you. Failure is too closely identified with disappointment, and we can have none of that.

Whoever you are I'm thrilled that you are expanding and investing in the process of fitness and health through real exercise and real nourishment. The weeks, the months and the years will go by. You know well enough that time gone by cannot be recalled or replaced and you'll not waste or abuse it. With these reflections, pursue your goals, envision and live the good days ahead. As time passes you will become more rather than less.

## Exercise, the dynamic that controls

- *Exercise done badly works better than no exercise at all.*
- *Exercise done half-heartedly works half as well as exercise done with desire.*
- *Exercise done occasionally does little.*
- *Exercise done regularly does much.*
- *Exercise done to please others is work.*
- *Exercise done to please yourself is joy.*
- *Exercise done in private is deeply rewarding.*
- *Exercise done with friends is bonding.*
- *Exercise done to kill time is time well spent.*
- *Exercise done to start the day is enormous.*
- *Exercise done to end the day is consoling and healing.*
- *Exercise done to raise the spirits never fails.*
- *Exercise done because you must builds discipline.*
- *Exercise done to calm the storm empowers.*
- *Exercise never done is a great, great loss.*
- *Exercise: Don't expect permanent or healthy weight loss without it.*

I am again reminded of the survey I did (page 28) and the 150-some odd responses I received in the first week. The email that filled my box was not from people completing an application form for another credit card or a quarterly tax return. The people were warm-blooded, emotional and passionate seekers who strained to answer confrontational questions. They admitted the project was a challenge and were grateful for the rough ground they were asked to cross. Their answers and the honest tone in which they were expressed gave me a dimension of reference I could not do without.

The only participants who were successful at achieving permanent weight loss and who exclaimed relief, joy and confidence were those who added regular resistance exercise to their life-long regimen of smart eating. They were once troubled and now stood out like brightly colored wildflowers in sun-parched fields. Where a majority fumbled with diet and menus alone, the successful participants applied action and energy and thrust.

The key is exercise. Accepting that fact is good. Embracing it is far better. Practicing it makes the big difference.

Where do we go from here? You tell me, and I will follow with suggestions. How about the beginning? Early on, a couple hundred words into Chapter 4, I applied mild pressure to get you into your sneakers, out the door and into a vigorous walk. This is the oldest and most reliable method to begin the exercise process and prepare you for more productive and specific exercise that builds muscle and strength and burns fat. I like spontaneity and recommend you practice the free-spirit approach on occasion to stretch your comfort zone, feel the rush and identify its power. As the guy who peddles gym shoes suggests, *"Just do it."* Breaking a non-constructive pattern is like tossing out the garbage. We need to do it regularly to prevent building up a pile in the backyard. Your goals have been revisited and page 28 has been reviewed. Get the body in motion and we'll go climb the mountains.

## Push that iron

Exercise, sweet exercise, the backbone to achieving a fit and appealing body—and who doesn't want a fit and appealing body, a healthy, vital and energetic system to carry on the business of efficient and joyful living? The reason people around the world don't embrace exercise and fitness more fully is because they don't understand it. It's lost in our culture; it's fading or it's reserved for the elite. The great human being, God's creation, in all his cleverness appears to be diminishing.

# Freedom

*Good morning, friend, and get outta bed,*
*Run 'round the block, you've got fat to shed.*
*Push that iron and lift that steel,*
*Who you are is how you feel.*

*Exercise is life's surprise.*
*Within its hold longevity lies.*
*We're not to say, "Some other time,"*
*To procrastinate is a gross human crime.*

*Consider the loss in vitality and desire,*
*As the body fails and systems misfire.*
*Sets times reps with focus and pace,*
*Intensity with sweat should you embrace.*

*This isn't a hardship, a pain to resist,*
*It's the thing of life upon which we subsist,*
*No nuisance is this, no curse to retire,*
*It's a thing of life upon which we aspire.*

*Give up the couch some time each week,*
*Walk, run, lift weights these goals to seek.*
*You're not alone and need not despair,*
*The fun's ahead and the game is a dare.*

The passages above would be particularly moving if read by James Earl Jones to the theme of "Rocky." Hold on to the seat of your pants.

There are as many ways to train as there are fingerprints and, at any given time, they will all work. Some work better than others, some forever and some only as a short experience to record that they are not valid for you.

You'll find that workouts from the onset can be stiff and uncertain. Relax. A few minutes past "Go" and a well-being and purposefulness surface, and you're rolling. Count on the aerobic exercise of your choice to warm you up and set you in motion.

# Biff & Mill

A couple came to the gym not so long ago looking like a pair of middle-aged porcupines in a field of wolves. I stood close enough to say, "How are you?" but not so close as to get a quill in my sweats. After I assured them that I wasn't there to sell them a membership, or mug or mock them, they relaxed and pointed out that they weren't interested in building massive muscular bodies. "We simply want to get in shape for the summer and our 20th high school reunion in July." He eyed the menu hanging above the juice bar and ordered a Jucy Lucy with extra mango extract. She fussed with her pantsuit that was beginning to gather around her thighs, "Where's the pool and hot tub?"

I stood my ground and contemplated the typical and sad catastrophe before me. No pool or hot tub to be found, I suggested that perhaps they consider a more aggressive approach to getting in shape by applying sensible weight training and sensible eating for the next month… or the rest of their life. Her name was Millie and I think she actually hissed under her breath. Biff was content scanning the gym floor and slurping his hefty protein drink. He thought out loud that maybe the weights were the way to go. "We could hire a personal trainer for a few weeks and learn the ropes, dear." She frowned and took a gulp of his drink, then another and another. She drained the 28-ounce plastic cup and tossed it.

We have a selection of aerobic equipment neatly laid out on an L-shaped balcony with plenty of height, light, viewpoint, breeze and TVs. This pressed Millie's button (treadmills, climbers and such… civilization), and I promised Biff a training appointment the following morning at 10 a.m. They both were relieved when I offered them a free week, giving them a chance to try out the ole shoe to see if it fit.

"There's something you need to know," I called out as they headed for the door of escape. (We made it. Well, almost.) I walked over and looked them directly in their eyes. "What you are mildly undertaking this day is probably the most significant *responsibility of your lives: your physical health and welfare. We grow up and grow older and watch from a safe distance. Today you've decided to participate. You're going to love this. Get a good night's sleep."*

They showed up early—their day off—revealing a humility and reserve undetectable the day before. New sweats, gym bags, sneakers and water bottles—matching bookends ready for a marathon. I greeted them and we headed for the bikes without preamble. A 10-minute warm-up before crunches and leg raises was the order of the day. I remained with them and told them about high-intensity interval training and promised we'd be doing that shortly to accelerate their progress. In five minutes the sense of involvement was achieved and they began to feel loose, sweaty and comfortable.

It turns out he had recently been diagnosed with adult onset diabetes and she had been... er... sort of binge eating regularly. They'd been married for 10 years, with a small thriving business in the convulsive industry of computer engineering—stress had a stranglehold on them. They were overweight, under-muscled, weak and vulnerable. They were brilliant yet ignorant. I think they were lonely. They were riding the bikes and smiling, and I was filling them with propaganda. The goodwill conspiracy.

Crunches and leg raises on floor mats were less of a delight, but they endured like champs. We hit the gym floor and decided that the Hammer Chest Press for shoulders, chest and triceps mixed with the seated lat pull for back and biceps was enough for one day. After three sets of 12 reps, pushing and pulling alternately, they were pumped and pooped. Hey! It was their first workout of a tired and mishandled lifetime.

Here's to commitment, discipline, courage and fear. They come in four to six days a week around sunrise to get a giant step on the world stress-makers and spend some exhilarating time with new, like-minded friends. Millie eats the right foods in the right amounts (often good nutrition accompanies good training) and Biff no longer takes medication. All the symptoms of diabetes are gone.

# Chapter 18

## Aerobics, Fat Loss & Muscle:
### *Sufficient vs. Excessive*

Weight lifting does not stand alone. Knowledgeable coaches compare the achievement of fitness to a stool of three legs: weight training, diet and aerobic exercise. Each leg must bear its fair share of the load to ensure balance. Who am I to disagree? I just accentuate the thickness of the weight-training support, establish a sturdy dietary leg and use aerobics as a balancing pole to maintain an upright, on-target position. I prefer to lean on hard, well-paced lifting and consistent, clean, high-protein, low-carb eating to set and control my muscle-building, fat-burning, cardio-respiratory health and metabolism with a side order of intense cardio to zero in on my course. Here I stray from the crowd. Physical fitness is vitally important. Aerobic exercise to achieve it, I fear, is overrated, over-consumed and over-worshipped. This doesn't make it bad. The "iron" is better—that's all... honest.

Aerobics come in all shapes and sizes from a brisk early morning walk to an all-out, indoor, interval-cycling class. Make your choice based on time, needs, goals, equipment availability and desire. Some folks love the high, the rhythm, the demand, the discipline, the socializing and the results. Jump in. But, please, don't let the activity become excessive or it may eat you up. There are, of course, those who absolutely hate the thought of running in place, the stationary bike and classes. If the thought of aerobics keeps you from the gym, forget it. Maybe some other time. Get in and get a weight workout.

Too much cardio will cut into your precious exercise time, available energy, training desire and focus. The model for aerobic efficiency is three or four, 12 to 20-minute sessions of treadmill, stair, bike or road work at varying levels of intensity each week: interval training. Here, the choice of modality is up to you according to desire, effect and convenience.

The amp in our fuel-burning system, engendered by aerobics, continues to burn calories for hours. Herein lies the real benefit of aerobics: ongoing fat burning via the chemistry change brought about by the exercise, when appropriate and smartly practiced. The calories burned during the actual running and jumping, kicking and screaming are minor. It's during this activity, over time, that the body creates enzymes important in fat-burning that carry on their delightful role long after our aerobic exercise has ceased for the day.

## Cardio training:
## Getting in shape or getting in trouble

I have a problem with the getting-in-shape approach to fitness, health and well-being. It carries with it a temporary connotation, as if getting in shape is something you casually gain and lose on a regular basis. Here today, gone tomorrow and here today again... more like here today and gone for good if you don't watch out. Make health and fitness a lifestyle and you'll shine like the bright summer's sun every day.

Bulletin: Eat right and exercise regularly. Smaller meals more often, more protein and fresh vegetables and fruit. Yeah. Yeah. Aerobics till I drop... Uh, uh. Wrong. Big wrong. Boy, have I fought this concept of physical fitness with a sword and a shield for years. Run, jump, dance, step, spin, jog... more, more... you're going to evaporate. Stop all that cardio nonsense and apply it with logic and intelligence.

Does this ring a bell? In the mid-'70s when the mainstream was first turning on to fitness, somebody came up with the running craze; lotsa carbohydrates to fuel the running machine, marathons, 10Ks, 5Ks, cardiovascular rules, run, run, run, burn fat, kill calories. The books and the doctors said so. Fit or fat, aerobic enzymes, classes on the hour; run, Jane, run. We became fully indoctrinated, programed, hypnotized—sold. The world of industry, commerce and big bucks took the cue and built the machines to keep us hopping. It, like Ford and BMW, continues to invent new gizmos each year and streamlines the old ones. Cardio training is big business. Cardio is overrated. Cardio needs to be sent to the back of the room like a spoiled brat and taught to behave according to our healthy needs. Bridle the frantic creature and make it work for you.

Seems as if the whole world forgot about muscles, protein and lifting weights for a quarter of a century. Twenty-five years of frustration has led us, thank goodness, to some very sound thinking and dandy cardio procedures. High-intensity interval training (HIIT) is a salvation for those determined to improve cardiovascular health, burn fat and spare muscle, sanity and time. Let me explain some basics.

Conventional cardio performed on equipment (bike, stepper, rower, etc.) consists of 30 to 45 minutes of even-paced activity. The participant seeks his or her preferred heart rate (by calculation or a heart monitor) and goes for the duration. The goal is to burn fat calories as well as develop the efficiency of the heart and lungs, the cardiovascular system. The activity raises the metabolism, and calorie burning continues for an extended period of time throughout the day. This works to a degree. Beats the couch, TV and a bag of chips by a miracle-mile. However, the monotony, non-creativity, invested time and scramble for equipment takes its toll on most everyone I know.

As a gym owner, manager and slave, I shudder, mop the gym floor and polish the mirrors furiously instead—the extent of my aerobics. It's very practical and it works. I love barbells.

Most recently—though convention is like glue—experience, experimentation and research are introducing smarter aerobic procedures. As soon as the training population gets unstuck, they might very wisely be installing HIIT into their fat-burning cardio regimen. Forty-five minute, low-intensity, long-duration sessions can be replaced more effectively with high-intensity interval training for an exciting 12 minutes. Yes, frazzled and delirious friend. There's life beyond treadmills and StairMasters.

Here's a simple HIIT sample for the free-spirited aerobic bum: Choose your weapon (spinner, treadmill, climber, outdoor jog or run) and plan on 12 minutes of output.

Of course, you're in suitable condition for the trial run, right?

Start an easy warm-up for four minutes, stepping it up comfortably as the minutes progress. I suggest you be in fair cardio condition before knocking off the 12-minute program. It can sting.

Body in motion and number-one endorphins engaged, you now blast it (according to your dynamite stores and desired explosion) for 30 seconds and back off for 30 seconds; blast it for 30 and back off for 30. Repeat this 30/30 interval session for a total of six sets or six minutes. The last two minutes are reserved for a gradual decrease in intensity and cooling off. You have completed your aerobics for the day. You expressed and challenged yourself, startled the dozing muscles and welcomed the sweet pain of gain. Boredom dwells with mediocrity, enemies not worthy of our company. Let's hit the weights and build some muscles. Race ya to the bench press.

You think I'm loony, joking or conspiring, don't you? Me not speak with forked tongue. I'll save you the dreary proof and challenge you to try the basic outline above and observe your activity response. You'll react hotly to the short-term extreme demand, and logic will convince you that intensity is setting new systems in motion. Creativity is welcome as you feel your way around the intervals. Vary the intensity load and rest intervals according to your moods and needs. Too few of us allow ourselves creativity. Cut loose.

Short blasts of high-intensity cardio snap the trainee out of the adaptive "steady state." The body wisely seeks to conserve energy (calories) when practicing the same-pace, low-intensity, long-duration protocol of ordinary aerobics. Tricks are in order. The metabolism reaches a more-heightened state for a longer period of time after high-intensity intervals, assuring the performer of continued fat-burning effects. Cardiovascular conditioning is achieved much sooner according to studying physicians.

Take the high road, feel the action, see the sights and get where you're going quicker.

# Chapter 19

## Getting Started:
### *Early Stages of Home & Gym Training*

Here's some advice from a former garagehead for those getting started at home with limited equipment. Everything within the pages of this book applies to you. You, with the right attitude and plan, will reach an exciting level of fitness, no doubt about it. Give yourself enough room to move freely, breathe and grow. Your private space and limited equipment can work in your favor. You develop efficiency in movement, a focus on the essentials and establish a bond between you, the action and the concepts of training. You will trim down your overweight body, shape it and tone it. It just takes time, persistence and a keen personal agreement to do it. Do you have these elements? Absolutely.

For starters, define your workout area: garage, spare room, basement—whatever. Neatly and concisely set up your equipment. What equipment? Ah, yes, there's that.

You'll find a lot of used equipment for sale if you want to shop the classified ads in your local newspaper, visit the flea market and garage sales or a Play It Again Sports (used sports equipment) store near you. Ask around. You might pull out the yellow pages and look under sporting goods and see what merchants are in the neighborhood. Larger cities will have major stores that specialize in resistance-training gear and offer impressive displays demonstrating the possibilities.

Let your enthusiasm, pocketbook and designated area guide you.

Start with the basics, which include a bar with enough weight (100 to 150 pounds to provide a variety of plate sizes for the barbell and your dumbbells, and for weight adjustments), a pair of dumbbell handles and a bench with racks. Build as you decide what you need and want.

Be a happy bodybuilder; hang a couple of posters and tune your radio to your favorite sounds for some cool background music. Atmosphere and a little company are always welcome. You're in charge, and you're getting close to the power source.

Give yourself 30 to 60 minutes, three or four days a week, to work out and, most importantly, set a regular time for this special occasion. Regularity is essential in establishing a mental identification, a "mindset," and in creating a physical pattern. Applying order from the very beginning will develop the strength of habit and give substance and discipline to your new undertaking, this matchless and life-changing sport.

Do things haphazardly and you get haphazard results. You'll miss the fun and fulfillment of completing a tough, focused and intelligent workout. You won't pump, burn, sweat or thoroughly overload. No endorphins, no natural chemistry improvement. Sooner than later, without foundation your inspired endeavor will fade to a guilty memory. Sounds dismal, doesn't it? Gets worse... your nose grows, your hair falls out and you can no longer squeeze into your super-large sweatpants.

Now what? Practice order and stick to the plan, Stan.

In the early stages, your job is basic. Practice and get to know your muscles, which muscles are working during each exercise and what are the factors of resistance, pump and burn. This requires and develops patience, focus and concentration, three amazing qualities to add to your list of accomplishments. You might make notations of the weights you use, the reps and sets, and a comment or two on a pad as a quick reference from workout to workout. This weight-lifting stuff is pure and simple, bearing your personality and standards; it becomes a vital extension and reflection of you.

You're a home trainer and ready to go. You've got your water bottle at hand. Hydrate and keep hydrated. A pre-workout meal with a balance of protein, carbohydrate and fat will provide fuel for energy and muscle restoration. Begin your routine by working your midsection for five minutes before hitting the weights. This activity will strengthen and define the trunk muscles, raise your heart rate and core temperature, stretch your muscles and engage your focus for the intense workout ahead. Several sets of floor crunches and leg raises to maximum reps should do it for now.

So much for the potatoes; now for the meat: the fun stuff, the major muscle builders, the big guns. There is no fast way to build muscle, get strong and lose fat; only hard work, good food and a lot of time will do that. Right? Right. There are no secrets. There are 50 exercises, maybe a hundred that we can choose. I've chosen the best to do the job for you. More is not better. Different is not better. Not today.

## Pouring the cement, laying the foundation

The plan is simple. I've listed seven favorite exercises and you are going to concentrate on those over the next five weeks to develop your skill and understanding of muscle and strength building. Refer to Chapter 20, Exercise X-rays, for an explanation of each movement. They are the basics and construct a sound foundation of muscle balance to give you years of dynamic performance. You are now going to practice and perform three sets of each of the following primary exercises:

## Primary exercises:

**Midsection—crunches and leg raises**
**Bench press**
**Barbell curl**
**Deep knee bends (dumbbells in hand)**

# Secondary exercises:

*Add one exercise per week:*

**Pullover with dumbbell**
**Bench dip**
**One-arm dumbbell row**
**Calf raise (dumbbell in hand)**

List the exercises on a pad, and make notes of the weight used and the sets and reps performed. This can be a temporary function to remind you of the details and serve as an initial focusing device. Your notes might look like this:

Midsection—
Crunches (2 sets x 25 reps)
Leg raise  (2  x 12)

Bench press (3 x 12), 100 lbs

Barbell curl (3 x 12), 45 lbs

Knee bend (3 x 12), body weight  (or with dumbbells)

Record keeping comes naturally to many trainers and is an invaluable tool in tracking and encouraging progress. If it works for you, your own methodology will evolve. It's not uncommon to see a professional logging notations in a well-worn volume as thick as an encyclopedia that he guards with his life.

# You look lost

Your job is to get the job done well. That means reading the brief description, practicing the exercise with all your heart, allowing awkwardness to pass and error to slide. One of your aims is to discover how much weight is appropriate for each exercise. The standard approach is to warm up with a light weight for a set of 15 repetitions. In the subsequent sets, add weight till a set of 12 repetitions is an agreeable force; that is, one more rep might be too many, one less rep too few. Record your choice and stay with that weight as you continue to practice and mature in the workouts to follow.

It won't be long before you are ready to increase the intensity with which you train. Once you are comfortable and confident with the early exercise resistance, once you've safely pushed and pulled with all your strength and the sets and reps are performed with precise form, it's time to add some weight to your bar. In the early stages of training you are free to feel your way around your new activity and become familiar with its dimensions. Your repetitions might go up to 15 per set to achieve the fatigue that 12 reps at first afforded. This is good and you are gaining understanding. Now you are ready and able to add weight to your bar and drop the repetitions back to 12... or 10. Try this alteration, see how it feels and go from there.

Soreness and stiffness are common and a natural response to the novel load of exercise on the ligaments and muscle insertions. These signals keep you aware of your limits, but are not meant to frighten you into a corner. Each workout calls for a warm-up period as we prepare our sometimes-grouchy muscles for hard work.

Muscles are better prepared for heavy force than their bone-attaching tendons, and it is often the unconditioned tendons that present initial pain or injury. Your first three to four weeks are a conditioning process for the entire system that has longed for your attention. The heart, lungs and vascular system are enriched by the new muscle overload. Much of the initial strength increase you enjoy will be from improved neuro-muscular pathway articulation, not an increase in muscle size. You're getting in shape to take on your environment, dominate it and lose those unwanted surface pounds. The timing could not be better.

Doing the job well calls for you to be entirely present during your workout. You can slide on through, thinking of a hundred other things, but you'll miss it, you won't get it, you'll be in the dark and you'll be sorry. Prepare for your workout by "psyching up" as the time nears, recalling your purpose and visualizing your goals. You have an hour, three days a week. Empty your mind and focus on the exercises, their proper execution and the muscles involved throughout the range of motion. Appreciate the work and the struggle and how to affect the particular tracking of the weights. Most people don't have the courage or foresight to lift weights, a tough and toughening challenge. You're a hero.

Note the pump (blood filling the working muscles for support and flooding them with oxygen and nourishment) and the burn (localized "hot-sting" produced by lactic acid, a metabolic byproduct that accompanies muscle overload). These two popular phenomena are signs of successful exercise application and the more you achieve of each the greater your training gratification. The more gratification, the harder you train and the greater the results; the greater the results, the deeper the commitment, the longer the investment and the more weight you lose, permanently; and you're back to gratification and so on and so on...There's more, and it keeps getting better. I promise. Wait till the endorphins hit. You are being indoctrinated.

## The structure develops

You are reacting, responding and adapting in innumerable ways as your body and mind absorb the impact of training. We talked earlier about the dramatic exercise-induced external and internal co-functions, the visible and the invisible benefits, and the synergy of their activities (hormonal activity, muscle density providing oxygen absorption and fat burning, etc.). You are prospering with compounding interest, and your investments are young.

The idea behind progressive resistance training is to increase the workload on your muscular system slowly and regularly through the manipulation of exercises, resistance, pace and various training techniques. The basic methods are discussed in these pages and will take you a long way to accomplishing your admirable goals.

You've already gone through phase one by adding weight to the bar. Next, one month into your start-up routine, you continue by adding one exercise a week for the next four weeks from the secondary list. Two or three sets of each movement further develop a practical network of muscle fibers, stimulate muscle tone and the metabolic processes, and prepare you for more aggressive training techniques. The joys of living, renewing and producing are sweeter than Tupelo honey.

I'm proud. You proud? We're proud. Not arrogant or conceited, just proud.

## Supersetting for reinforcement

Long ago when man was groping about the misty and craggy surface of the earth he stumbled across superset training, an intense and energetic style that broke away from the stale, single-set strongman methodology. I was an early proponent who carried forth the principles with resolution, and today I center my workouts on them as I perceive them as unfailing.

Much of what I've learned has come from observing people in action on the gym floor, an extraordinary cross-section of people training with purpose and good intentions. Today as I look out over the gym's square footage, observe the variety of activity and listen to the range of questions thrown my way, I'm convinced that flow and continuity in training should be encouraged from the very beginning. Once a new lifter completes the first weeks of introductory exercise and gets a feel for the equipment, muscle resistance and his level of condition, he is ready to practice interesting exercise combinations that piece the workouts together. This style of training is called "supersetting," when two or more exercises that complement each other are performed one after another before resting to enhance lifting output. This multi-set training not only condenses workout time, it also increases productivity considerably.

Single-set training—resting after each exercise set—has its place in your workouts and should be retained for strength and mass building. However, a training scheme blended with superset combinations adds excitement and dimension to your daily routine. A highly gratifying and inspiring muscle pump is achieved as blood, laden with oxygen and tissue-building nutrients, fills the individual muscles, causing greater muscle growth.

Supersetting is a technique I've applied for more than 40 years (gulp), one I put into use long before reading a muscle magazine or going to a gym. I instinctively gravitated toward a non-stop training style to maintain enthusiasm and momentum. Without the downtime between sets, I become more involved in my training. There's no time for daydreaming or boredom or wishing I were somewhere else. In fact, a most desirable attitude of *training* develops, one that we wrongly associate only with athletes on the edge of competition. This perception of *training* is a valuable tool of confidence and provides a very real psychological benefit for a straight talker like you.

With a little time and a little practice your training becomes more athletic as you move from one exercise to another. Your heart rate remains higher, you stay warmer as you near the edge of aerobic training, your concentration becomes locked and the harmony of movements lures you onward.

I'm often asked why I superset. Because I like it. Because I like the pace, the rhythm, the flow, the accelerated perfection of form, the athletic feel, the etching repetition, the dance, the busy-ness, the involvement, the pump, the burn, the efficiency, the cardio-respiratory application and the high. I notice I'm able to add hard muscle as I eat smartly. I'm able to employ a more-complete percentage of my muscle tissue with a locomotion of sets and reps performed with exact full range of motion, intensity and zeal. My first rep is thoughtful and deliberate; my last rep is thoughtful, deliberate and red-zone intense. The volume delivers maximum-force saturation, maximum muscle involvement. I'm a slave.

## The ground floor

You are woman. You are man. You are ready.

You have one solid hour for each workout according the the weekly schedule. Now that you're six weeks into your training foundation, give yourself loads of time for your new workouts to determine your level of condition, familiarize yourself with your surroundings and exercises, and enjoy the novelty and substance of your new endeavor. Clear your mind and be attentive to the task at hand. Any sense of pressure or anxiety, unless directed toward your workout, will be counterproductive.

Ease into your new workouts with two or three sets of each exercise. Increase the number of sets to three by the end of the second month, with your eye on four.

These beginning programs use the superset technique. There's no rush; practice your movements at an agreeable pace with confidence.

The simplicity and order of these routines is contagious. The novelty will lure you into your early workouts as you practice and learn the exercises. It won't be long before a sense of understanding and accomplishment take over and the rhythm and flow of exercise are experienced. This is comforting and becomes a motivating aspect of weight training that only the attentive participant will recognize. I mention this quality now so that you might seek it and enjoy it sooner, as opposed to letting go too soon and not enjoying it, ever.

# Routine 1

**Midsection exercises and warm-up:**
Crunches (1-2 sets x 20 repetitions)
Leg raise (1-2x10)

**Exercises 1 and 2, done together:**
Bench press (1-4x12, 10, 10, 8 repetitions)
   *superset with*
Stiff-arm dumbbell pullover (1-4x10)

**Exercise 3:**
Partial stiff-legged deadlift (1-4x8-10)

**Exercises 4 and 5, done together:**
Barbell curl (1-4x8-10)
   *superset with*
Dips between benches or chairs (1-4x10-12 or maximum)

**Exercises 6 and 7, done together:**
Light bar squats (2-4x15)
   *superset with*
Calf raise off block (2-4x15-20)

# Routine 2

This is an ambitious addition to the first routine and is intended to demonstrate a variation of program expansion. You can compare the two sample routines and blend the two as you choose. Additional exercises are listed to expand your selection and enlarge your boundaries.

When changing routines or making alterations, allow extra time and be prepared for experimentation, consideration and delay in training flow.

You might at some point purchase additional weight, an extra bar and dumbbell handles for convenience and workout efficiency. Should home training appeal to you, the investment is well worth it. You'll be ogling squat racks and pulley systems before your birthday, Christmas or the next tax refund.

It's not unusual for enthusiastic trainees to join a gym and split their training between home and commercial facilities on a regular schedule to enjoy both atmospheres. The luxury of having the option is obvious; suit your mood, suit your timetable.

Use the same abdominal warm-up. This function will gain in its priority as you continue with your progress and discern your needs. You've got one hour, four days a week—an extra day with extra interest and willingness. You can now apply the split-routine technique: upper body (torso) on day one, arms and legs (extremities) on day two, rest on day three, upper body on day four, arms and legs on day five, days six and seven off, and repeat the following week.

# Days 1 & 4
## Torso

Bench press (2-4x8-10)
   *superset with*
Pullover—stiff-arm (2-4x12)

One-arm dumbbell row (2-4x6-8)
   *superset with*
Dumbbell press, low incline (2-4x8)

Dumbbell shoulder press (2-4x10-12)
   *superset with*
Lateral raise, bent-over (2-4x8)

# Days 2 & 5
## Arms and Legs

Curl, seated dumbbell alternating (2-4x8)
   *superset with*
Lying triceps extension (2-4x12)

Barbell curl (3x12-15)
   *superset with*
Dips between chairs (3xMax)

Squat (2-4x15-20)
   *superset with*
Calf raise (2-4x15-20)

Deadlift (2-4x8)

You'll find the exercise descriptions and a list of routine variations in the upcoming pages, beginning with Chapter 20, page 193.

# Reassurance

As you get familiar with your routine and workout area, it will flow and become comfortable. Be attentive and confident. There's nothing to doubt. You're doing absolutely the right thing at the right time. Stick to your outlined routine for at least six weeks with growing intensity and assurance. Only then will your body adapt to the consistent overload and build muscle. During these days you'll practice, develop form and learn a hundred things I can't describe, things you'll discover that will add to your life more than you ever expected.

If you don't play hard and work hard in your daily life, plan to add aerobic activity to your schedule three days a week for 12 to 20 minutes. This will, of course, increase your fat-burning, muscle-building metabolism and improve the health of your heart, lungs and vascular system. All this combines to enhance your energy and endurance to train more effectively.

With a month or two invested in your new workouts you'll be familiar with the elements of training and the responses of your muscles. You'll be conditioned and ready to increase your resistance output. These routines, with gradual weight and repetition upgrades, can serve you successfully for six to eight months. Does it appeal to you? Stick with it. Are you ready for a change? Move on.

Early trainees are often impulsive and impatient. They change routines too soon or too often, before either good habits or healthy muscle have a chance to develop from consistent and thoughtful overload. Don't succumb to premature training changes due to improper assessment or no assessment at all. Hang in there.

## How to choose a gym

A resourceful young lady restless with her body's fitness collected and clipped together a selection of my weekly email newsletters. She gleaned through the contents and extracted the thoughts and strategies that appealed to her. Furthermore, she applied them—at first in an awkward way— and discovered to her surprise an internal ability to connect the chaos I offered and found a working continuity as she practiced. She hung to the words "determination," "persistence" and "patience" until they became more than words but her very own budding attributes.

"I've changed," she says, "I'm ready to go to a gym." Good for her. It takes courage to seek out a gym and walk through the front door expecting a throng of obnoxiously confident and shapely bodies to evaluate your hips and biceps. Your nifty home gym in the garage, basement or bedroom becomes most attractive suddenly, limitations and all. You miss your favorite blue mat and the clunk of your dumbbells. Relax. Let's pick out a gym for our daring friend and talk about her choices. Let there be light.

Gyms come in all shapes and sizes: squares, rectangles, L-shaped, U-shaped, upper level, two stories. Go to the cities and they're on penthouse floors; go to the suburbs and they cover acres, with ball courts, pools, restaurants and golf facilities. Each gym has its own personality largely based on its ownership and operating team, the neighborhood in which it resides and, subsequently, the folks it attracts. Like a mate, there's a gym for everybody.

Here's a summary of determining factors to consider, and how they might suit your expectations:

- **Price**

A usual first consideration, but how much it costs to get the most of what you want and need should not be at the top of the list. Hopefully you'll recognize the imperative nature and true value of your training activity and decide that you'd easily pay more for a gym that inspires.

- **Location**

The nearer to home, work or the center of your activities, the better. The world has become complicated and excuses fly when we're on the wrong side of town. Time is money. Right? Truth is, there's no excuse to put your health and well-being in second place to getting home or even going to the bank. Convenience is golden. However, don't let it dictate joining a gym you find unlikable just because it's at your offramp.

- **Hours**

Here's where 24-hour gyms shine. Just knowing you can go anytime you want has a great appeal. Where do you fit in? Try your best to set a time when your minutes in the gym are honored, unrushed and efficaciously applied. Smile. Be happy. Will you really train at 3a.m.?

- **Phone contact**

Let your fingers do the walking for the first curious steps. If you dial a likely gym and the gym employee snaps, "What do you want?," you might put a little question mark by that name and go on to the next facility on your list. If you ask price and the answer becomes a secret, put a check by that name and move on. Slick talk is not reserved for carnivals and used-car dealerships. We have to be sharp. Listen for honesty as you engage in conversation, whether professionally conveyed or offered through inexperienced youthfulness. Eventually you'll want your answers made clear in a visit and a week's worth of complimentary workouts.

- **Member volume**

How crowded does your prospective gym get? This is a major consideration and can be determined only by visiting the facility at those hours when you'll normally train. Hop on a stationary bike for a 15-minute cruise and assess your surroundings. What if this was your home training ground? A grand gym down the street with all the attractions and equipment is of no use at all if you can't work out with focus and efficiency because there are too many bodies on the floor. In fact, the anxiety that ensues is a near crisis to the serious trainer. You want to move smoothly from exercise to exercise without mobs, glares or testy attitudes. Hey, is there parking?

- **Amenities**

Don't pay for a lap pool, giant sauna, lounge and aerobics room if you're not going to use them. More is not necessarily better, and it might be necessarily more expensive. Larger gyms tend to be clubby. Is that what you're looking for?

- **Equipment**

The quality and condition of equipment and the choice of the tools of the trade are central to the final decision. Well-maintained, seasoned machinery—not fresh out of the crate—can be more useful and fun than the recent trick gadgetry turned out daily in this big-bucks industry by tacky, techy entrepreneurs. Enough equipment is enough; too much, poorly laid out, can be a setting for a factory and not an appealing, functional gym.

- **Atmosphere**

Are you standing in a muscle-building gym or a scene where boy meets girl and they hang out like it was the mall? Do the babes cheer the big guys as they spear their Olympic bars across the floor and grunt? Do you think this is cool? No? Go to the next merchant of fitness on your list.

- **Management attitude**

Look for respect, politeness, honest and direct answers, and an eagerness to show you around to discuss your needs and the gym's attributes. Do you feel like a number, a dollar sign or a fellow iron-and-steel aficionado? It happens not infrequently that a good gym is the victim of the bad rap that comes from the bottom-line sharks uptown and several minutes of open conversation brings the dross to the surface.

- **Clientele**

Who's to your left, who's to your right and can you stand them? Are they snobs; are they slobs? Do they yell, groan and bang the weights around? I'm bad. Do they tiptoe, wiggle and whimper? You want to feel comfortable, accepted, appreciated and encouraged where ever you are. You want to look forward to your time in the gym when you can focus, learn and grow. A good gym should be a refuge where you can lick your wounds, as well as a haven of energy for hard work and physical expression.

• **Cleanliness**

Cleanliness and neatness are two outstanding qualities that define the ownership and membership. They are marks of order, responsibility and respect. Perfect is not possible where people by the hundreds work and play, but a unified effort to keep the corners clean is admirable, to say nothing of hygienic. Let's put our weights away and pick up after ourselves, encouraged the merry ole muscle maker in a jolly voice.

Happy hunting.

## So this is a gym?

The gym is across the street, and the time has come. You're a big girl (or should I say a big boy?), but you wish this part were over. You've made the phone calls, and your fingers have done all the walking they're going to do. The rest is up to the feet and the big chicken stuck to the other end.

First time to the gym, is it? I can't tell you what to expect because every gym is different depending on the community, size, style and the ownership and staff's personality. You've narrowed it down according to location, convenience, word of mouth and the trusty phone calls. Very cool. And the free pass is at the front counter waiting for you as promised.

Move the feet and enjoy the experience. You've got work to do. You want to get past the strategic front counter with finesse, eyes, ears and smile fully engaged. Once on the gym floor, practice your walking, breathing and relaxing. Attaching yourself to a stationary bike for 10 minutes will give you a safe perch from which to observe and prepare your next stunning maneuver. Also works well to warm up the body, get those neuropathways activated and start distributing endorphins. They calm you, kill pain and generally make you feel better.

There is nothing more pleasant than a pleasant gym member. There is nothing more obnoxious than an obnoxious gym member. Here are some hints to keep you in the right category:

• Look for any posted rules and observe them. These might be common courtesies, time regulations regarding aerobic equipment, carrying a towel or limiting the use of fragrances.

• Be aware of the space around you. Equipment and bodies are forcefully moving in different directions. A crowded gym can be a red zone. Do not whack anyone in the head or other body part with a dumbbell.

• Replace barbells, dumbbells and plates in their designated places after using.

• Carry only the gear you need with you and leave your gym bag in a safe place off the floor or in a locker. Prevent clutter and hazard.

• The age of leotards has passed with Sputnik. You can relax and train comfortably in sweatpants or shorts, a T-shirt or sweatshirt.

• Proper footwear is important for your health and performance. Pick up a pair of your favorite Keds at the mall and reserve them for your workouts. A smart gym won't allow street shoes, sandals or open-toe footwear on the gym floor.

• A towel to keep you and the equipment you use dry is a smart idea. Good hygiene is very popular.

• A breath mint, when necessary, is a crowd pleaser.

• While we're on a roll, fresh gym clothes and deodorant never disappoint anyone. However, excessive fragrances will turn up noses, and body oils are gooey.

• Don't commandeer any piece of equipment; accept that people might want to share in its use. Sharing equipment is called "working in."

• Nix on forcefully clanging dumbbells or dropping the weights.

• Excessive noise in exerting force is less popular than some people think. Boisterous conversations and raucous behavior is disturbing to the majority. Be cool.

You're doing just fine. Oh, by the way, your sweats have a hole in the bottom.

# Chapter 20

## Exercise X-rays:
### *Descriptions of Exercises*

You've arrived. Menus you have read by the dozens, copied, torn from pages of magazines, folded and shared, praised and scorned. Nothing new about eating, and diets are as old as the hills. Barbells, dumbbells, cables and squats, however, are possibly a departure from your daily routine. Let the novelty lead you by the hand and the worth of the activity carry you along.

As we move to the exercise descriptions, I'll describe them in appropriate detail throwing in bodybuilding talk as I proceed. I ask you for latitude in presenting the muscle material to maintain the sense of its native performance. I fear over-articulation will produce over-trying and stiffness in approach.

I've opted to communicate in a conversational tone throughout the book, as that's the language most of us understand and with which we are comfortable. I apply that tongue in the exercise descriptions to follow. Baby talk or teacher-like instruction suffocate the adventuresome attitude of training I hope to convey. Let's not treat the bench press and curl as if they were brute aliens; let's embrace them like future old friends, loyal and supportive.

Need I remind you that form is of primary importance? Form is followed by focus, and pace, and then immediately by the weight used. This does not minimize the importance of the weight used; it simply guarantees and accentuates the value of sure performance.

Every exercise suggested in the forthcoming routines of *Your Body Revival* is listed and described in the following pages. Read them over to gain a fundamental understanding of the movements and further your insight into the curious iron game. Plan to personally supply a barrel of practice and logic, an ounce of curiosity and a shot of risk, the inherent ingredients for establishing meaningful workouts.

I've also composed a short list of terms and their definitions common to the weight training scene. They might prove useful and interesting. You'll find them in the glossary on page 245.

# Exercises—the list of 38

Bench press
Cable crossover
Calf raise
Crunches
Curl—bar, dumbbell, EZ (bent) bar, machine
Curl—preacher or Scott curl
Curl—seated dumbbell incline
Curl—seated or standing dumbbell
Curl—thumbs-up, hammer curl
Deadlift
Deep knee bend
Dip—freehand or triceps press machine
Dumbbell fly
Dumbbell press
Hanging leg raise
Hyperextension
Lateral raise—bent-over
Lateral raise—front, hammer plate raise
Lateral raise—side-arm
Leg curl
Leg extension
Leg press
Leg raise
Lunge
Lying triceps extension
Military/overhead press—clean and press
One-arm cable crossover
One-arm dumbbell row
Pulley pushdown
Pullover—stiff-arm or straight-arm
Rope tuck
Row machine
Rubber tubing—rotator cuff work
Seated lat row—low pull
Squat
Stiff-legged deadlift
Wide-grip pulldown—front and back
Wrist curl—reverse wrist curl

## Bench press

The bench press is one of the patriarchs of weight training and one of the three lifts in the sport of powerlifting, a family whose siblings are the squat and the deadlift. This comprehensive movement builds a network of upper torso muscles including, primarily, the front deltoid (shoulder), the pecs (chest) and the triceps (back of the arm).

Lying on your back, grasp the racked bar with a grip some six inches wider than shoulder width; press overhead with a slight arc to a neutral starting position directly over your shoulders. Once you've momentarily established and briefly held your starting position, lower the bar slowly and deliberately (known as the eccentric or negative motion) to the bottom of your chest. Allow the bar to make full contact with the body before immediately reversing the motion and pressing the weight to its original starting point (the concentric or positive motion). Smoothly repeat until your designated reps are achieved.

Focus on the muscles involved, carefully guiding the bar through its range of motion until you discover your groove—the exact track for the bar's movement according to your skeletal-muscular mechanics. Allow one or more seconds to lower the bar and power up steadily after reaching the chest. Practice—there's no failure at this stage, only correcting and re-correcting, trying your best and improving. You'll personalize all your exercises as you grow, perform, learn and understand.

## Cable crossover

Cable crossovers are not a power movement, but they are significant in shaping and defining the entire pectoral region. Stand in the center of the apparatus with the cables in hand. Take a giant step forward and, with semi-stiff arms but elbows bent, draw the handles high and straight forward, leaning as you do to counterbalance the resistance. Continue with a full range of motion, extending and contracting evenly and deliberately. Upon completion of the contraction, reverse the motion with equal resistance to a wide-armed, stretched, starting position. Repeat. Focus on upper pec contraction for six reps until the burn is considerable, then shift the handle movement to a

45-degree angle toward the floor. This engages more pec mass allowing you to force out another four to six reps. Vary the angle of movement according to fatigue and to target different ranges of the muscle. Seek rhythm, flow and tight contractions.

Cables drawn high across the pec recruit upper chest muscles near the clavicle, tying them in to the front deltoid; the lower the action, the lower the pec musculature recruited. I prefer single-arm cable crossovers to further the range of motion and direct the resistance more accurately and with greater muscle-building contraction.

## Calf raise

Standing, toes on an suitable block, simply raise and lower your heels to engage the calf muscles. Resistance is achieved by bearing weight across your back with a bar or via a machine, or by holding a dumbbell in hand as you stand on a block applying one leg at a time to the task. Alternatively, the donkey calf raises are performed by leaning forward on a supportive object and having a partner sit across your back as you raise and lower off the by-now-popular block. There are machines that allow you to sit while resistance is applied to the calves in a bent-leg position, thereby shortening the calf muscles and directing the effort to the soleus (alongside and under the calf muscle). Mix them, supersetting seated with standing, for example, as you devise your routine.

## Crunches

Lie face up on your favorite bench or piece of floor, knees bent with feet shoulder-width apart and pulled tightly toward you. Position your arms behind your head and cradle your head in your hands. From this stable starting place, with a minimum of tugging on your head, roll your upper torso forward into a C-like posture, your upper back rising off the floor as the abdominals contract to complete the movement. Maintain your focus on the muscles involved. This contraction should be split-second, yet super tight—the peak of muscle overload and adaptation. Slowly lower yourself to a full and deliberate starting position and repeat for sets of multiple reps.

A weight plate can be held behind the head or across the chest to add resistance; lower the reps if using the plate. Right and left obliques and intercostals (muscles on the side of the torso) are recruited as we slightly twist and lead with the right or left elbow as if reaching for the space between the knees. Mix them up, for example, 20 to the front, 10 left, 10 right and 10 front, totaling 50 reps for one set. Getting warm, oxygenized and movin'—I call this the "super crunch."

Crunches tone and strengthen the entire abdominal area with an apparent emphasis on the upper region. They provide maximum muscle action with minimum expended energy. Mild crunches are a therapeutic exercise and safe on the lower back, a good introductory exercise for the willing-and-able obese, elderly, injured or beginner. Good stuff.

### Curl—bar, dumbbell, EZ (bent) bar, machine

A curl is a curl is a curl? I don't think so.

I do all of these movements regularly and enjoy them equally. The straight bar works well unless rotation at the peak of the movement torques the wrist and the ache of strain limits your input. (This is where a thick-handled bent bar comes to the rescue.) Stand erect with your feet shoulder-width apart and the bar hanging fully extended before you. Pull the bar somewhat in front of you and up at the same time to a point even with the shoulders. Pause only long enough to reverse the action and lower the bar slowly to the starting position.

Your reps in all exercises will vary according to the muscle, its mass and fiber, and your goals and scheme. I work reliably in the six-to-10 rep range, matching my mood, endurance and level of repair. As I fatigue, and this is evident in all my training, I draw upon a calculated body thrust to enable the completion of the final tough repetitions without losing workload integrity. These deep, hard reps call the rest of the body to action. As long as they are defined and directed, they'll work for you.

These are big, full-biceps builders if that's your target. None better. The heavy curls with built-in thrusts put a welcome demand on the system, shifting from single-joint isolation movements to broad-range muscle recruiters. Dig in.

Machine curls are like compact cars; they're designed to get you from one place to another. Drive one, you can drive them all; it's just that some are a better ride. Hop in, wiggle till you're comfortable and pull. Now you've got it. I'll be over here doing dumbbell alternates. Don't fall off.

### Curl—preacher or Scott curl

The preacher bench is that apparatus that looks similar to the lectern you'd expect a preacher to stand behind, his bible and other reading material afixed to its angled top. You know the drill: You approach the bench when it least expects it, sit down like you are going to take a breather and then suddenly and fiercely wrap your legs around the thing, grab the suspiciously close bar and start curling in hungry reps over its padded and perfectly angled surface. Some people claim tendinitis from the outward slant and prefer to curl from the reverse side of the padded slope, which allows the arms to drop straight down; no hyperextension, no elbow aggravation and no over-curling to stress the brachialis (upper forearm muscle). Instead, lots of intense, isolated biceps pulling and slow, vascular, mind-altering descents. Let someone else count if anyone's keeping score.

### Curl—seated dumbbell incline

Choose your favorite incline angle (experiment until you find it) to give your biceps the extension and mechanical advantage you desire. Stay tight, let the dumbbells hang, then pull them, palms forward, toward the shoulders; contract and slowly lower. Same old curl, yet different enough when you fight the metal going down to the count of three or four, rep after rep; or curl them outwardly from a super-extended, palms-out position, up and down like fire and ice.

### Curl—standing or seated dumbbell

Let's see. How does it go again? Assume either the standing or seated position with the dumbbells hanging by your side, fully extended and palms forward. Just as you would in the barbell curl, pull the weights slightly forward and up to shoulder height. Don't do anything fancy as if it would make a difference. Pulling the weight with all you've got is sufficient. With each new rep, focus all your attention on the movement of the weights, the path they travel and the team of muscles aching, pumping and burning to finish the rep. Notice the change in demand as the dumbbells are lowered, stretched and taut, to the starting place. Note the relief that comes with the pause, the drawing in of air and the tightening of the body as the mighty process is repeated until it can't be repeated again.

### Curl—thumbs-up, hammer curl

A variation of the curl that I've been doing since an injury 15 years ago that urged me to stray from the norm, the thumbs-up curl is an exercise twist that I've come to know quite well. Stand as indicated earlier, only now the dumbbells are held palms facing inward. Here again, drag the weights upward but in a slightly modified groove, one that brings the plates toward the face—the cheekbones, to be precise. This positioning clearly puts a demand on the forearm and across the biceps, a welcome and productive diversion.

Moreover, I, who seek water from a rock, find that with a mind on the back muscles, front delts and minor pecs, this movement with explosive-yet-controlled thrust and emphasized negative hammers nearly the whole upper body. Sets of 12, 10, 8, 6, 4 supersetted with wrist curls and pulley pushdowns are common with me, just to be sure.

### Deadlift

Deadlifts are a simple exercise really, made difficult by over-trying and over-thinking. Stand before the weight in a solid, shoulder-width stance (or up to six inches wider), shin to the bar. You are about to bend over and pick up a heavy object, and this should be your mental approach.

Bend at the waist and at the knees equally and at the same time. Grasp the bar fully and securely, with an over-grip or in an alternate under/over-grip, about waist width, hands just outside your legs. Looking straight ahead, your spine in a powerful flat position (not stooped over or rounded), focus, breathe deeply and steadily pull the bar to a full, standing position. Keep the bar close to your body and exhale as full force is exerted. Pause for a second of contraction and slowly bend your knees and low back as you return to the starting position. Repeat.

Two to four sets of 10 reps, twice weekly with a light to moderate weight, should be of substantial benefit during your first six weeks to condition the many muscles involved, and to discover form through practice and the possibilities of application to your goals and system of training. A safe placement for this exercise is at the end of your leg workout, as it complements quadriceps work, or at the end of your back work. Seventy-percent output should suffice in the early stages to set the foundation, build muscle and prevent training overload and injury. It takes time to prepare the thigh, hip girdle and erectors for heavy powerlifting.

The day will come for many when the urge to lift a maximum weight from the floor to your waist for a single rep will challenge you. Be ready—wisely done, deadlifts that approach triple, double and single reps after warming up are exciting and productive. Exceedingly heavy workouts done twice every four to five weeks are a valuable addition to your training regimen; you'll experience systemic muscle growth and an increase in overall core muscle and power. Workouts producing personal records (PRs) are truly memorable.

Women who seek to strengthen, shape and tone their buttocks, hip and thigh areas will respond well to this formerly all-male power movement. A comprehensive and stabilizing exercise, deadlifts should become a standard practice throughout your years of training. They will produce most-agreeable changes in your shape and performance. Throw in squats and you'll be delighted.

Don't hesitate. With care, daring and proper instruction, you can humbly boast of their presence in your scheme. Finally, only practice and experience will teach you.

## Deep knee bend

Here's an alternative to the barbell squat that can be performed freehand (without weight) or with a pair of dumbbells hanging at your sides. Standing erect with your hands on your hips or extended before you for balance, lower yourself into a deep knee squat position while maintaining an upright upper body posture. Feet should remain flat on the ground throughout the exercise, and you should push off from the lower-most point through the heels of the feet to the upright

starting position. That's one terrific rep. Three sets of maximum repetitions where 20 is your limit will serve you well. Do this exhilarating
exercise (large muscle-work places a high demand on the cardio-respiratory system, the heart and lungs) twice or three times a week as
you progress.

Practice the movement to condition the thighs, glutes and the
connecting leg muscles. If needed, hold on to a stationary object (power
rack, chair back) in the early stages to control balance. Soon you'll be
able to perform the action with light to moderate dumbbells in your
hands, lowering the repetitions and putting more resistance on the
muscles involved.

The deep knee bend with moderate to heavy dumbbells is an
interesting replacement for squats when change is desired or an excellent substitute for the squat when using a bar is not viable (inadequate
equipment or space, or, perhaps, tenderness across back and shoulder
regions). Practice and focus on groove and muscle action develop this
athletic movement into a formidable addition to any workout. The
added resistance in the grip and through the arm, trap and back areas
is a great benefit to the body's muscle and might. Sets ranging from six
to 15 reps are productive.

### Dip—freehand or triceps press machine

Wide-grip dips, a.k.a. wing-whackers: Lean forward, round the
back and direct the effort toward your mid-back via partial reps. The
more you lean forward and the deeper you go, the more the chest
muscle activity. The narrower the grip and the more you totally lock
out your elbows, the greater the triceps effect. Freehand bar dips are,
of course, more demanding and potentially more mass-producing than
regulated machine dips. You will not be practicing these for some
time to come, though some weight-loss champions have made freehand chins and dips part of their successful goal package.

Machine dips allow resistance control, muscle targeting and partial range of motion when limited by injury. When I first learned how
to walk, I padded over to the kitchen chairs, arranged them back to
back and began to perform dips. My mom had to count out the reps;
my math was weak.

## Dumbbell fly

Flys are executed to engage the pectoral muscles in their most complete and isolated action by drawing the extended arms across the chest. They are performed on the flat bench or any intelligent degree of incline or decline. Assume a position lying on your back with a pair of lightweight dumbbells overhead. Maintain a near-straight-arm arrangement, palms facing each other; lower the 'bells outward until they are in line with the body (or parallel with the floor); pause and return with willful pectoral contraction. Bone structure, insertions and muscle mass frequently determine the effectiveness or success an exercise has on a person. Consider this: The upper arms tend to dominate the execution of the fly, and the movement thus does little to shape and define the pecs and lots to shred or tear the biceps. Your job, through focus, is to direct the resistance (the weight load) to the chest muscles. This takes practice and concentration, two ingredients which define good training.

Flys make for a terrific burning and pumping secondary movement in a chest-pressing superset.

## Dumbbell press

Whether done on a flat bench, decline or incline—even an upright shoulder press bench—this is basically the same mechanical movement. Simply put, as the flat-bench-press position engages the center-chest mass and front deltoid, the incline shifts the resistance to the upper-chest mass and demands more shoulder; the decline conversely gets lower pec and minimizes deltoid involvement.

Sit on the edge of the bench with the dumbbells, plate down, on your lower quads. Draw the dumbbells to your waist as you roll back to a lying position, immediately thrusting the weights up to an overhead starting placement. Palms forward and elbows outward, lower the weights to the sides of, but not quite even with, your head. Power back up to the start, take your pause and repeat. Practice, seek your groove, focus and you're on your way.

Dumbbell presses are a better and healthier exercise than the barbell bench press in many ways because the hands can rotate to accommodate the needs of the frequently overused and abused rotator cuff or shoulder device. The barbell bench press is rigid and unforgiving. Also, with 360 degrees of direction in each hand there's a need for a lot of muscle stabilizing and coordination, meaning more demand for muscular health and growth.

Dumbbell inclines are the favorite big-deltoid builders of pro bodybuilders over the years. A 45-degree incline up to 75 degrees is a nice range of variation for the years to come. Muscling your dumbbells into place is also a structure- and skill-building process. Don't drop them and don't clang or crack them at the top. Control them. Be nice.

### Hanging leg raise

The ultimate in leg-raise effort starts by hanging from an overhead bar with your hands. Hang and, with slightly bent legs (or legs bent a lot—it's easier); raise your legs upward to some "doable" point of contraction; then lower again to the starting point and repeat.

Easy, until you start swinging out of control as the rest of the gym watches in amusement or horror. The hanging leg raise takes a little practice and should be introduced once the trainee is conditioned and confident. The trick is to fast forward the reps (up, down, up, down, without pause) to prevent a pendulum action from developing. I dare ya.

Incidentally, this is a great exercise for building grip and upper torso hanging strength.

### Hyperextension

An important exercise for lower back development and stability, the hyperextension is performed on a specific piece of equipment. Hyperextension benches differ one from another, but the mechanics are the same. You eventually find yourself lying face down across the apparatus, the back of your lower legs held firmly to support your upper body which is extended outward from the hips and down in a starting placement. Slowly raise your torso upward and approach a horizontal or straight-body position, hold the contraction for a second and lower in a two-second count. Short trial movements will prepare you for and familiarize you with this unlikely exercise. Your ascent is slow and thoughtful, cautious not to come up too fast or too far, distressing your lower back. Hypers are more agreeable than they sound, and their back-protecting benefits are invaluable. Twice a week for three sets of 12 to 15 reps nicely complement a midsection routine. You know what they say, "A man or woman with a strong back lives a lifetime."

### Lateral raise—bent-over

Stand before a pair of iron knuckle-busters. Greedily pull in some oxygen, with the back of your hand wipe the sweat from your brow, bend over and firmly grasp the dumbbells. Bend your knees and rest your ribcage as best you can on your quads to protect fatiguing erectors from overload. Allow the dumbbells to hang, palms facing each other. Pull the dumbbells high and outward to a position even with or above your flattened back. Contract the rear delts, concentrate on the negative return and repeat. Go two reps per breath. Done.

Rear deltoids (the back of the shoulder), though relatively small, are very appealing in appearance, powerful in performance and important for healthy mechanical balance. The muscles, however, are insufficiently trained, and they require specific exercises to recruit them. These exercises are awkward and limited in range of motion, thereby relegating them to the bottom of the preferred exercise pile. Doesn't make 'em less important.

### Lateral raise—front, hammer plate raise

This is my version of the front lateral raise. Most of what I do is tainted by time and injury, not that I'm a hundred years old or falling apart. Just a few almost-pleasant limitations encourage me to modify and sometimes eliminate a few of the movements of my trade. This solid, counter-pose, plate grip "fixes" my shoulder and enables front-delt action I would otherwise be unable to enjoy.

Sitting on the edge of a bench, feet planted but with legs extended and spread out for stability, grasp a flat plate with both hands and allow it to hang, ready for the first rep. Easy.

Raise the plate with locked arms, directing the resistance through the hands and onto the front deltoids. Peak resistance is achieved at a point some 45 degrees above horizontal, and rotation beyond this range becomes a risk. Lower to the starting position using the eccentric properties of the exercise to load the delts. Feel the compressing action of the grip in the pecs, the upright thrust within the traps, the peculiar demand on the straining biceps, and the muscular stabilizing throughout the back and torso as they fight for balance. A light weight serves to warm up the rotator cuff; heavier weights with a thrusting motion can be serious. Don't underestimate the dinky stuff.

### Lateral raise—side-arm

This ever-popular dumbbell movement isolates the outer head of the deltoid; it shapes and completes that which presses begin. The best way to learn the exercise is to start with a pair of very light dumbbells hanging by your side a little to the rear of your body, palms facing inward. With the arms slightly bent at the elbow, raise them outwardly to a position just above parallel above your shoulders, palms down. Repeat the movement for a set of 10 repetitions, and notice how cleverly we modify the action to reach our goal as we fatigue: a teeny lean forward, an imperceptible bending and shortening of the arms, a mini-thrust and a crossing of the eyes. Fact is, you're on your way to the perfect side-arm lateral raise to give your deltoids practical strength and assertive presence.

Don't stop now. Work up the rack, eventually, and improve your form and thrust with tight contractions at the top and negatives that complement the strengthening action. Who said these isolated, simple movements are simple and isolated? Get rolling on these shoulder makers and you have heavy breathing; lower, middle and upper back working in concert; grip work and some random parts of the outer biceps burning. Are you intense? Superset side arms with seated press behind neck. Original in '62.

### Leg curl

The leg curl is a machine exercise that works the muscles on the back of the thighs—the hamstrings—also known as the thigh biceps. Typically an under-worked muscle, the thigh biceps should be brought into balance with the quadriceps to provide overall strength, protect the leg complex from injury and add appealing symmetry to the body.

Position yourself according to the mechanics of the apparatus, adjust carefully and perform the reps as indicated. Three to four sets of eight to 15 reps twice a week work well. I seek tight contraction and commonly do curls as the second part of a leg-extension-and-leg-curl superset, doing single-leg calf block stretching during the pause between supersets.

## Leg extension

Performed with the assistance of a machine, the leg extension works the powerful four-part muscle structure of the front thigh called the quadriceps. It has its place in the training of the thighs, though I reserve it for the first part of my leg extension/curl/calf-raise tri-set. This demanding union placed before my squat workout serves as a significant warm-up and heavy-load preparation. It strengthens and shapes the quads, yet I am reluctant to apply more than a guessed 80-percent last-rep overload as a caution against knee risk. Remembering adjustments for personal needs, I do five sets of 12 to 15 slow and steady reps with moderate weight, no momentum and a brief mid-rep contraction. Lactic acid exudes; fire everywhere.

## Leg press

We're stuck on machine work here, aren't we? Though quality, efficiency, comfort and load bearing roam a wide range, all leg presses are basically the same. Sit down, secure your feet on the platform, make yourself comfortable, unlock and press. Secret: A good leg press works a lot better than a bad leg press.

Foot placement makes a big difference in targeting development or engendering an injury. Feet too close or too low on a platform often result in knee abuse. Legs angled too far out or placed too wide (uselessly hoping to recruit adductors to trim loose flesh from the inner thigh) cause pain and damage as the natural knee tracking has been severely compromised under stress. A common sense, shoulder-width, natural toed-out footing that is thoughtfully high on the footplate will provide the safest and most productive arrangement to power through your muscle-building reps. Pushing through your heel and traveling slowly through your reps and sets will maximize their affect. Don't go too deep at the bottom of the action or you'll eventually cause a muscle tear or hip, low-back, knee or ankle stress. Makes ya grouchy.

## Leg raise

Leg raises can be performed on the floor or off a flat or 10-percent inclined bench. They're tougher than crunches, working more of the lower ab, groin area and hip flexors. They also present antagonism to the hips and lower back if attention to your body mechanics, positioning and form is not sensitive. According to your readiness, I suggest you extend your arms totally forward and place your hands comfortably under your tailbone. This platform and counter-posing, upper-body muscle action relieves, if not entirely eliminates, low-back pressure, as will bending the legs slightly at the knees. Now you can rep out with only the abdominals and hip flexors crying out in muscle-building pain.

The action starts with the greatest intensity from the floor or bench as your extended legs are slowly and laboriously lifted to a near overhead, thigh-perpendicular position. Up and down with a moderate pace governed by the good struggle, you are applying yourself to a classic favorite. The awkwardness diminishes as the workouts go by and you enjoy their benefits. I sound like I'm selling them by the pound and today is the last day before they go bad.

Your reps may not exceed 10 or 12 as the hip flexors and muscles of the groin region seldom bear direct resistance. They'll be sore tomorrow; don't flip out. Once I thought I had appendicitis; another time a hernia. Turned out to be a rep too many on a muscle too weak.

## Lunge

I prescribe lunges for a stretchy, pumpy movement between sets. That's all. Then again, Laree likes 'em a lot more. She does them off a raised platform, protecting the knees while offering a more complete and targeted range of motion. Sisters of steel may want to experiment, making the prime target the glute and hamstring tie-in.

## Lying triceps extension

Lying on a bench, grasp a light barbell or bent bar with your arms extended overhead in a narrow (six-inch) grip. Start the triceps extension by lowering the bar to your forehead or further beyond your head. The upper arms are to remain elbow tight and upright to emphasize the load on the triceps and guarantee maximum development. The triceps extension is a major mass and power builder. High reps pyramided with low reps (and a heavier weight) work well to saturate the three-headed muscle.

The overhead triceps extension performed similarly from a seated upright position (wisely using a utility bench for back support) with the elbows straight overhead is another aggressive triceps builder. The employment of the bent bar is a popular alternative. Remember, tendinitis prowls. Warm up; don't overload excessively.

## Military/overhead press—clean and press

Standing or seated, this is tough. Grasp the bar just outside shoulder width and position it across the front of the shoulders just under the chin. It will require some practice, trial and error to pull the bar from the floor in one swift and directed motion to the target starting position.

Hint: Partially bend over and partially squat down to grasp the bar and then, with focused might, pull the bar up to the shoulders and allow the weight to cradle on upturned palms and front shoulders. The power comes from the concerted effort of the thighs and back. This is an amazing exercise all by itself which is called the power clean, part of an Olympic lifter's clean-and-press exercise. It's a very comprehensive movement for dynamic, overall structure development and explosive power: lots of traps, low back, hamstring and quad. A favorite of serious football players for the kind of explosive power needed to crush the opponent. Fun stuff.

Once in place across the shoulders, press the bar continually to a locked-out overhead position, briefly hold and slowly lower to your shoulders and repeat. This is to be done with a minimum of back lean or leg thrust. I highly recommend you use a tough leather lifting belt to girdle the midsection and protect the lower back.

This is not a low-level or medium-level movement. It is a high-level movement, comprehensive and systemic, meaning in simple terms a full-body, major-muscle and multi-joint exercise, responsible for sending messages throughout the entire body to grow—to adapt—to meet the demand. This includes enzymes, neural pathways and hormones.

Nevertheless, this movement can be beneficially installed in your routine early on, once you've established a working understanding of exercise and your physical condition. Cleans and presses are super for fat loss and muscle growth.

## One-arm cable crossover

The one-arm cable crossover beats the dual-arm in that you can give superior focus to all ranges of pectoral activity, achieve a greater range of extension and contraction, work one side at a time with maximum output and modify the action to incorporate surrounding, hungry muscle groups: serratus, lats, and biceps.

Position yourself alongside the cable apparatus as if you were about to perform a typical two-hand cable crossover. Crouch slightly in a position of readiness and, with shoulders remaining in a straight line with the cable system, draw the single handle with an unyielding straight arm high across the pecs. Back and forth, contract, extend, contract—look for rhythm, continuity, flow and burn. As high-pec muscles fatigue after four reps, drop to a stronger mid-pec hand-and-cable groove 45 degrees toward the floor before you. Another four reps, then finish with a shift in body to bring the cable directly down toward the floor as you locate low-pec recruitment.

Have fun with this rangy exercise: improvise, feel, isolate, customize. Make it yours. Back and forth.

No supersetting here; apply this combination to the end of your chest routine, three to four sets of 12 reps, one side followed immediately by the other. Form, muscle location, isolation and burn are everything.

## One-arm dumbbell row

This potent exercise stands with barbell rows in mass and power-building seriousness. Executed with the same intensity, they are wisely done as alternatives to the barbell. Stabilized in a powerful tripod stance—none of this knee-on-bench stuff—one-arm dumbbell rows remove the load from the lower back, enabling you to tough your way through lumbar overload. Relief in this overworked area is priceless.

I stagger my legs, bend at the waist and lean on the dumbbell rack before me; extend my free arm to grasp the dumbbell, position myself for desired muscle recruitment and pull the weight toward the body in a muscle-intense movement with an ample twist of the torso at the top to accentuate contraction. Too much thrust early on and the effect is lost to momentum. The target of the tug is important: High on the torso (toward the shoulder) uses more upper back; low on the torso (toward the obliques), more lower lat.

## Pulley pushdown

Not a power or mass exercise, the pushdown effectively forms the triceps and adds to their health. Grip your favorite handle and stand approximately a foot away from the overhead pulley. Bend your arms at the elbows and bring them close to your torso, directing them slightly forward. Extend the handle downward to a straight-arm position, contracting the triceps tightly. Slowly return to the starting point with an accent on the negative for maximum advantage. I regard the pushdown with affection and apply ample body thrust to load the triceps totally while properly engaging an army of associated upper-body muscles (erectors and torso stabilizers, serratus, minor pec and upper back). This vigorous performance transforms the minor isolated action into a more substantial movement packed with energy and spirit. Ideal for supersetting with biceps curls or a major triceps exercise applying sets of 12 to 15 reps.

## Pullover—stiff-arm or straight-arm

Performed with a barbell or a dumbbell, it's a "feel good" power stretch that engages the lats and the underside of the biceps, triceps and chest muscles as it puts the rotator cuff through its range. Longitudinal abdominal muscles come into play to stabilize the torso. Did I mention they build the serratus like the mason builds walls of stone?

If you like supersetting, a stiff-arm pullover between sets of almost anything is gratifying and productive. A moderate weight allows you to stretch, revives the muscle cells and adds immensely to upper latisimus building. Keep the secondary pullovers at eight to 10 reps.

Lie on your back, head on one end of the bench, feet on the other end and grasp a dumbbell or barbell in your hands straight over-head—your starting position. Take a deep breath as you slowly lower the weight behind your head with stiff arms, elbows nearly locked. When your arms are in line with your torso—parallel to the floor— reverse the motion and return to the starting position, exhaling as you do. Pause momentarily and repeat. It's a great stretch, great lat pump and a great relief movement that promotes posture awareness. Lots of blood circulating oxygen and nutrients to wake up, stimulate, revive and refresh.

Let me clarify the hand positioning when using a dumbbell. Sit at the very end of the bench and place the dumbbell plate-down on your thighs. Place your wide-open hands on the inside bottom plate to the left and right of the handle. Draw the web of the left hand close to the short bar, fingers remaining outstretched and grasping. Mimic the procedure with the right hand, allowing the fingers to over-lay the left. Tuck the stabilized dumbbell to the midsection and roll back, thrusting the weight to the overhead starting position. Bingo.

### Rope tuck

This one's my favorite. The rope tuck, while specifically an ab-dominal exercise, can be manipulated by body positioning and concentrated muscle contraction to work countless details of the up-per torso. Start with a pulley system that provides a single overhead cable from which you can attach your favorite rope handle. Choose an appropriate weight through trial and error (approximately 30 per-cent of body weight), grab the rope, kneel down about three feet in front of the system and sit back on your heels. Bend forward toward the weight stack with the rope under tension and hands close to your lowered forehead. You're ready to practice the movement as you as-sess the resistance throughout your abs and the upper body and as you determine your range of motion and facility to move with muscle-focused efficiency.

The first 10 reps are performed with the arms held fixed, rope-grasping fists near your temples and the torso moving up and down by the power of the abs. Important: The entire abdominal muscle region is contracted to do the hard work. Don't lunge forward and accomplish the motion with the assistance of your body weight. Nice try.

Continue the action with a slight shift of the body to the right for five longer-motion reps, and, likewise, shift to the left and repeat. These variations add interest and further the involvement of the torso to include the obliques and intercostals (muscles along the side of the torso). An extended overhead range of motion affected by the cable enables you to bring in serratus and lats (swimmer's upper back muscles) while you are continually loading, stimulating and fatiguing the grip and biceps.

We've got the whole family playing, the heart's beating and the sweat's pooling. I don't usually stop there. We're 20 reps into the set and there's five or 10 or 15 left. Take five more tucks to the front to complete and balance the abdominal obligation. Then we pull ourselves off our knees and, in one motion, bring the legs around and assume a seated position, whereupon we allow the cable to completely extend forward; we're still on our haunches and savoring the relief of extension. The hands are giving way, but not until we count five more tugs with the rope to the front of our body, our chest and back arched and contracted. That's set Number One. I love to superset these with lightweight deadlifts for four sets of 10. Perhaps I can forego the aerobics today.

## Row machine

Adjust the weight, grab the handles, place your feet securely on the footrest and sit with your arms extended and under the resistance of the weight stack. The starting position has you in an erect, slightly arched upright posture as if elegantly seated in a straight-back chair. Lean forward slightly as the chest pad allows, pause and begin your motion by pulling back while simultaneously drawing in your arms. As you approach the ending position, begin to arch your back recruiting your mid-back muscles, further drawing in your arms to your midsection (just below your rib cage) to complete the movement.

There you are: seated upright, back arched and flexed, arms drawn in and flexed. Grand. Continue this terrific action that simulates the rowing of a boat for 12 to 15 reps. Practice and you'll find this will become an all-time favorite—most productive for practical strength and wonderful for muscular growth.

### Rubber tubing—rotator cuff work

The rubber tubing used in the following exercises is a length of springy rubber tubing approximately 54 inches long, available in differing tensions with handles afixed to each end. This simple apparatus serves us well to perform movements of a minor range, yet of a major importance: injury prevention, muscle therapy and on-the-road or at-home exercise.

Attach the free end of the tube to a fixed support (gym rack, hand rail or such) about waist high. Stand firmly with your working arm by your side, bent at the elbow. Resistance properly directed, rotate your hand inward, thereby achieving the therapeutic pronate action. Redirect the tube resistance and rotate your hand away from the body to complete the supinate action. Complete four sets of 25 smooth, high-paced reps of each action for both left and right sides as an upper body warm-up.

Five years ago this exercise combination was seldom witnessed at our gym and was considered for saps only. Today we have a dozen multicolored tubes of various tensions being pumped in every corner of the gym giving it the appearance of an amusement park. This movement is serious, deserves focus and 100-percent effort. It does wonders to develop the minor rotator cuff muscles and tendons that stabilize the shoulder and provide resistance and muscle fullness. The usual presses and laterals don't affect the shoulder straps and do require their loyal and tenacious support to help you blast away. Delts need to be warmed up and treated kindly. Perform these cuff rotations regularly to maintain health and achieve full deltoid potential.

### Seated lat row—low pull

The knees are out of the way and your favorite close-grip handle is extended as you reach forward. Pull the handle tightly toward the waist as you arch your back to contract the rhomboids, ending in an upright-seated position with a very slight, five-to-10-percent lean to the rear. Very nice; have fun with the purposeful negative. No thrusting, no momentum—strictly muscle, power and form. This can be supersetted with your stiff-arm or bent-arm pullovers if you like to keep your hands full.

These low pulls are a loveable exercise even when they're nasty. Nice positioning, energizing, cat-like stretching and extending, followed by might in the controlled contraction. The reliable 12, 10, 8, 6 sequence with intense muscle work, 55-mile-per-hour pace, tightly arched contraction, no pointless leaning back or dangerous, excessive forward lean. Mid-back and low-lat sweep are the direct targets of this all-time standard. Good for moms, their spouses and their kids. My dog likes this one.

## Squat

The squat is a comprehensive, full-body muscle builder. The full range squat movement adds strength and athletics to the entire torso more directly than any other exercise on the list. The accent is on the glutes (butt muscles) and quadriceps (thigh muscles). Unless you have racks from which you can retrieve the bar, you'll "clean" the bar (Remember? Hoisting it up from the floor) to locate it across your shoulders. This is no easy task and will result in the use of light weight for higher repetitions. Fine. Gives you the opportunity to practice your clean and press (a mighty movement requiring technical skill and practice) and get your lower back, knees and thighs well prepared for your future of heavy squats—a must if you can and will.

Bar in place across the traps and shoulders—padded if you choose with a folded towel—assume a natural, toed-out, shoulder-width stance. Oxygenize by drawing in several deep breaths and lower yourself as if you were about to sit down on a chair. The butt goes out and down; your lower back, hips and knees bend in concert. Down you go keeping your eyes straight ahead, bar steady and over your knees, feet flat until your thighs are near parallel to the ground. Up you go, pushing off with your heels. Be careful not to tip forward allowing the back and bar ascent to lag behind the leg thrust. Upright, take a deep breath and hold it going down, keeping the torso muscles tight. Upon reaching parallel, push up and exhale as you ascend. Repeat till the reps are achieved—one-and-a-half to two seconds down, one-and-a-half to two seconds up. You get it? You've got it. Don't try to walk up or down stairs for a day or two. It'll be ugly.

Early stages of squat practice and conditioning permit abbreviation of the movement until confidence and structure are developed. If you have the advantage of a squat rack with adjustable safety stops, set the stops to allow a one-foot descent. This range is sufficient for tough workouts and gives you the opportunity to train hard and build muscle, balance and familiarity. As your workouts advance you can lower the bar appropriately until you achieve your preferred depth. You've arrived. See deep-knee bends as an alternative if you're just starting out.

### Stiff-legged deadlift

A lighter variation of the bent-leg deadlift or powerlifter's deadlift, stiff-legged deads are practiced using relatively milder weight targetting the hamstring for stretch and flexibility and the resulting improved health, strength and performance. The full torso, lower back and grip benefit modestly as well. Standing upright on an eight-inch block with a slight bend in the knees and the bar in hands, palms toward the body, lower the weight to the floor. Look straight ahead as you focus on the descent, keeping the resistance safely close to the body along the shins to a near-ankle pause and steadily pull up; shoulders, back and arms extended and in control.

In the case of both bent and stiff-legged deads, at the moment of descent the backside moves backward as the lowering weight is kept close to the body (the center of gravity) in obedience to the laws of physics. Expect this logical compensation, and you'll find the movement more appealing and achievable.

Repeat for eight to 10 or 15 reps for the number of sets defined by your purpose and drive. This large action—like a piece of your own puzzle—fits where you want it.

### Wide-grip pulldown—front and back

To the front:

Positioned directly below the overhead pulley, legs held steady by the kneepad and arms fully extended, pull the bar to just below your chin as you look upward. Your back should be arched, your chest straining toward the bar with your elbows back, not forward, all positioned to fully recruit the entire latissimus complex—width and length.

Allow a sufficient lean and tug with no excessive thrusts to accomplish your well-formed reps. Don't cheat—no momentum. Feel, locate, pump, burn and grow.

As freehand chins may be absolutely impossible for you these days, by all means do the appropriate pulldowns to enable you to aspire.

To the back:

Use a medium grip and situate yourself slightly forward of the overhead pulley. From the fully extended starting position, pull the bar deliberately down directing the resistance to the upper back muscles, rear deltoids, biceps and lats. This is best achieved by concentrated isolation of this region by pretending you are onstage before the judges and are instructed to hit a back pose. Contract up and down smoothly, tightly, rhythmically.

Here's a longtime strategy I use to engage everything in sight: Tightly contract the upper back muscles as you pull the bar to the base of the skull for six reps. Use the negative return for full muscle recruitment—lats, near the scapula or wings of the upper back. Position yourself so there will be no need to dangerously thrust your head forward to allow the passage of the bar. Continue the final six reps to the chin as described previously with sufficient tug to overload the back. You're flying.

### Wrist curl—reverse wrist curl

Choose an Olympic bar for balance and smooth plate rotation; straddle a bench, grasp the bar with a complete finger and thumb under-grip and rest your forearms on your thighs for cushion and stability. The bar in hand extends just beyond the knees and is slowly lowered to a full and safe range, then curled back up to a tight, contracted position. This is done with slow, concentrated might to ensure maximum muscle growth and avoid wrist injury. After 12 to 15 reps, release the thumb and allow the bar to roll down the length of the fingers and partially curl again for a pumping and burning four to six reps. This mean tag team engages the complete hand, wrist and forearm mechanics.

To superset this with a reverse wrist curl, grab the bar with a hands-over grip, similarly place the forearms on the thighs for stability and logically perform the isolated, reverse wrist curl. This is an awkward movement with little muscle mass to recruit. A light weight with focus will efficiently add to your forearm's balance and might.

## Exercises by the truckload

We could go on and on. There are as many exercises as there are pounds in gravity. We've covered most of the good ones and I expect you'll invent some of your own. Every exercise has a dozen or more hidden inside it, which you discover as you lean this way or that, modify your grip or alter your footing, stand or sit, arch, bend or extend your torso, or straighten your arms a little or a lot. There's an angle and range of motion for every need. Be curious; discover and uncover them, make them yours.

# Chapter 21

## The Weights:
### *Training Routines—*
### *Introductory & Comprehensive*

The intention of *Your Body Revival* has been obvious: to persuade you to eat right and pressure you to exercise. I've tried every angle and every approach. I've no doubt angered, bored, annoyed, harassed, bewildered, hoodwinked or embarrassed you. I'm sorry. Well, not exactly; sometimes you've got be mean to be noticed.

And here you are—X marks the spot—the perfect place at the perfect time. A friend from our IronOnline.com website wrote me a note when I indicated nagging doubts about the need of yet another weight-loss book. He pressed me to complete the project saying that the continued input improves the probability that a flash of revelation or inspiration will finally strike a reader; the accumulation of information and encouragement force open the floodgates, or the manner in which an idea is presented gives it clarity and meaning at last. What I have written is not new or earth shaking. There is nothing new under the sun. Let's take comfort from that truth, and get to work.

I know the target from the outset and the general direction in which to aim the bow. I affix a handcrafted arrow equipped with a unique sensory device. I stand ground, and with all my might draw the string to its full extent and release, launching the arrow at a wide arc. It changes direction imperceptibly as it seeks the mark. Each day that I write I hope to strike a chord, ring a bell or fan the embers of desire, commitment and energy. I want to help. I don't need to hit the bull's eye; the tail will do.

In preparing the list of training routines, I questioned the wisdom of including advanced training techniques, the more brutal, full-throttle workouts typically reserved for well-seasoned lifters. The minus is I might chase you away, confuse you or inadvertently fool you into thinking such preposterous training measures are necessary. The plus is I would offer you a popular variety of possibilities from which to tailor your workouts for a long, long time. I chose the latter. They cost you nothing extra, and I preface them with verbal softeners to prevent you from beating yourself to a pulp.

As you proceed with your training, grab a copy of *Brother Iron, Sister Steel* for its more advanced twists and turns.

## Lift that steel

The following are model workouts for you to adopt to suit your preferences and your gym's equipment list. Unless otherwise indicated, I recommend that you continue your routine for four to six weeks before changing. Start with the Full-body Workouts 1 and 2. They are your basic training ground; study and practice them with patience and tolerance. When the time is right, go on to the variety of routines that are offered. Pick and choose among these—they're in no particular order—or make up your own. Be tough. You're alone with yourself. Become an encouraging, empathetic and upbeat training partner. No slouches allowed. Continue to be healthfully self-tolerant and self-loving, yet aggressive. Cruise for two or three workouts until the wheels are turning. Don't you dare stop now; it's a good ride.

*Full-body Workout 1*
*Full-body Workout 2*
*Upper-body/Lower-body Split*
*Quick-fit Program*
*Rotation Training*
*Draper All-time Favorite*
*The Time-crunch Equalizer*
*Leg Priority Training*

# Full-body Workout 1

Complete one or two sets of each exercise the first two weeks and three sets of each the remaining weeks of the four-week cycle. Be easy: During the first set, warm up and practice the groove of the movement, the track in which the weight safely, effectively and naturally travels. Toward the end of the cycle, increase the resistance with each successive set.

# Monday/Wednesday/Friday

**Midsection and aerobic work**
10 minutes of interval cardio, crunches and leg raises

**Chest**
Incline dumbbell chest press (x12)
Dumbbell pullovers (x12)

**Back**
Wide-grip pulldowns (x12)
Row machine or one-arm dumbbell row (x12)

**Shoulders**
Dumbbell shoulder press (x12)

**Triceps**
Triceps press machine or bench dips (x12)

**Biceps**
Standing dumbbell curls (x12)

**Legs**
Leg press or squats (x15)
Leg extension (x15)
Leg curl (x15)

Focus, form and deliberate motion. Work hard, but don't strain… yet.

# Full-body Workout 2

A few additions and a little shifting of exercises give this routine more variety and volume. You're up to two to three sets per exercise, 12 different exercises total. It's more time-consuming, but you'll be able to move more confidently, more surely and with less rest as your understanding and condition improve.

## Monday/Wednesday/Friday

### Midsection and aerobic work
10 minutes of interval cardio
Crunches, leg raises, hyperextensions

### Chest
Dumbbell chest press (x10-12)
Cable crossovers, pec dec or incline flys (x10-12)

### Back
Wide-grip pulldowns (x12)
Seated lat row (x10-12)

### Shoulders
Dumbbell shoulder press (x10-12)

### Biceps
Barbell curls (x10-12)

### Triceps
Triceps press machine or bench dips (x12)
Pulley pushdown (x12)

### Legs
Leg press or squats (x15)
Stiff-legged deadlifts (x15)
Leg curl (x10-12)
Calf raises (x20)

Some activists will scream that this is too much volume, but you're not yet blasting the sets, and you need the activity and practice. Volume is good (reps x sets x exercises per workout equals exercise volume). Your last rep of each set should feel just right, with near-perfect form and concentrated muscular action. Muscle burn—the sting within the muscle being worked—increases with each successive rep. It's a good pain which, when endured, allows greater muscle overload and subsequent increased muscle adaptation, therefore muscle growth.

Look for the pump, the full muscular feeling that is evident in immediate muscle increase during exercise as blood fills the muscle cells under demand of systemic support. The pump is a mighty good feeling.

This is another routine to be done following a four-week cycle.

## Upper-body/Lower-body Split

Time to split your routine; that is, divide your routine into two parts done on separate days: upper body on one day, lower body on the next. This intermediate system of training allows you to work harder with more enthusiasm and focus in a shorter period of time per training session. More muscle work is accomplished throughout the week with sufficient recovery time providing accelerated conditioning, fat burning and muscle development. The schedule you choose can accommodate your goals and weekly activities. Day one followed by day two, one day off; day one followed by day two, two days off is a commendable combination.

# Daily

**Midsection and aerobic work**
10 minutes of interval cardio
Crunches, leg raises, hyperextensions

Workout routines follow on the next page.

# Day 1—Upper Body

**Chest**
Bench press (3-4x12, 10, 8)
Dumbbell flys (3-4x12, 10, 8)

**Back**
Chins or wide-grip pulldowns (3-4x10-12)
One-arm dumbbell row (3-4x8-10)

**Shoulders**
Steep-incline dumbbell press (3x8-10)
Lateral raise (3x8-10)

**Biceps**
Bent-bar curls (3-4x8-10)

**Triceps**
Dips or triceps press machine (3-4x12)

# Day 2—Lower Body

**Legs**
Squat (4x12, 10, 8, 6)
Stiff-legged deadlifts (3x10)

Leg extensions (3-4x12)
  *superset with*
Leg curls (3-4x10-12)

Standing and/or seated calf raises (4x maximum reps)

## Quick-fit Program

Here's a 50-minute workout routine put together mainly for the in-a-hurry crowd ripping up and down the malls, highways and office cubicles. It's clean and neat, and, with thoughtful periodic exercise replacement, this outline has the concise and efficient appeal to last a long time. It's like dessert.

## Monday/Wednesday/Friday

15- 20 minutes of aerobic work

5 minutes of torso work:
Crunches
*superset with*
Leg raises (2x maximum reps)

Chest press—dumbbell, bench or machine (3-4x8-12)
*tri-set with*
Stiff-arm dumbbell pullover (3-4x8-12)
*and*
Row—any type of cable, machine or dumbbell
(3-4x8-12)

Barbell curl (3-4x8-12)
*superset with*
Triceps press or dips (3-4x8-12)

Leg press (3-415-20)

## Rotation Training

Rotation training provides freedom with control, order without conformity. It's as advanced as you want it to be, yet suits a healthy beginner if presented knowingly and patiently by an experienced partner or personal trainer. It's like stepping up to home plate and hitting doubles and triples your first day at bat.

## Day 1

Aerobic exercise, 15 minutes
Midsection work, 10 minutes

### Chest, Back & Shoulders

Bench press, bar or dumbbell (3-4x8-12)
   *superset with*
Wide-grip pulldown (3-4x10-12)
   *or*
Chest-press machine (3-4x8-12)
   *superset with*
Row machine (3-4x10-12)

Dumbbell incline press (3-4x8-12)
   *tri-set with*
Dumbbell pullover (3-4x10-12)
   *and*
Seated lat row (3-4x8-12)

Dumbbell shoulder press (3-4x8-10)
   *superset with*
Bent-over lateral raises (3-4x10-12)

As your conditioning improves, hit your favorite cardio hard and move directly to your crunches and leg raises with little rest between supersets. Twice a week throw in two sets of rope tucks and hanging leg raises. This fast-paced abdominal work maintains a high heart rate, thereby extending aerobic uptake. A great advantage, a gift. Pick one superset of the first two listed. The third combination is a tri-set that'll flow like lava.

# Day 2

Aerobic exercise, 15 minutes
Midsection work, 10 minutes

**Arms & Legs**
Barbell curl (3-4x6-12)
   *superset with*
Triceps press (3-4x10-12)

   *and/or*

Alternating dumbbell curls (3-4x6-12)
   *superset with*
Pulley pushdowns (3-4x12-15)

Leg extensions (3x15)
   *tri-set with*
Leg curls (3x8-12)
   *and*
Calf raises (3x20)

Squats or leg press (4x10-12)

Deadlifts (4x12, 10, 8, 6)

Bent-bar curls are comfortable and safe for the grip and wrist, yet a straight bar provides an unusual total biceps action and peak overload. Experiment, compare and creatively mix the two. Start from a full-arm hanging position and powerfully pull the bar toward your chin. A controlled body thrust or cheating-like action is okay in the heavier or fatiguing repetitions with a medium-to-slow lowering of the bar to the original starting position. A mighty movement that puts an advantageous demand on the whole upper torso—erectors to traps—it's a great multiple investment to complement Day One output.

To perform dumbbell alternate curls—standing or seated, doesn't matter—bring the right dumbbell from a palms-forward, fully hanging position tight to the shoulder with a medium-to-slow return to the straight hanging start. Add a mini-second pause, and repeat with the left. A little rocking, a little thrust, a little growling and you're in there. Follow this by your standard pulley pushdown done with might and form.

Leg extensions, leg curls and calves are tri-set counterparts. Deliberate, clean, piston-action reps get you through some painful lactic acid blues. Leg presses are safe, sound and productive if you don't roll your lower back by going too deep—tough on the knees and lower back. High reps (15-20) are most productive for early leg conditioning, toning and muscular advantage.

Add high-rep deadlifts for a strong back—a classic favorite of hardcore lifters with a generous heart. This is an excellent addition to a mundane routine. Gives it guts and charm; your choice.

## Draper All-time Favorite

After all is said and done, my favorite training routine is based on a seven-day week, three days on—one off, two on—one off, reaching a six-week stretch with enough daily wiggle room for comfort.

**Midsection—Torso**
Your favorite variation of crunches (incline and weighted), leg raises, hyperextensions, hanging leg raises

**Monday—Chest, Back & Shoulders**
Dumbbell bench press (3-5x12, 10, 8, 8, 6)
   *tri-set with*
Wide-grip pulldowns (3-5x12, 10, 8, 8, 8)
   *and*
Standing bent-over lateral raises (3-5x6-8)

Dumbbell shoulder press (4-5x12, 10, 8, 8, 6)
   *tri-set with*
Dumbbell pullovers (4-5x12, 10, 8, 8, 6)
   *and*
Seated lat row (4-5x12, 10, 8, 8, 6)

**Tuesday—Legs**
Leg extensions (3-5x10-12)
   *tri-set with*
Leg curls (3-5x8-12)
   *and*
Calf raises (3-5x15-20)

Squats (5-7x15, 15, 12, 10, 8, 6, 6)

Deadlifts (5x10, 8, 6, 6, 6)

**Wednesday—Arms**
Rubber tubing rotator cuff,  5x20
  (Each arm, in toward the body and away, 4 positions total)

Wrist curls (3-5x20, 15, 15, 15, 15)
  *tri-set with*
Thumbs-up curl (3-5x10, 8, 8, 8, 6)
  *and*
Pulley pushdowns (3-5x12-15)

Bent-bar curls (3-5x6-8)
  *superset with*
Dips (3-5x12-15)

Dumbbell alternate curls (3-5x6-8)
  *superset with*
Lying triceps extensions (3-5x12, 10, 8, 8, 8)

**Thursday—Off**

**Friday—Upper Body**
Overhead press (4x12, 10, 8, 6)
  *superset with*
Pulldowns (4x12, 10, 8, 6)

Dumbbell incline press (4x12, 10, 8, 6)
  *superset with*
Pullovers (4x12, 10, 8, 6)

Dumbbell rows (4x8)

Dumbbell alternate curls (4x12, 10, 8, 6)
  *tri-set with*
Dips (4x maximum)
  *and*
Pulley pushdowns (4x12)

**Saturday—Legs**
Same as earlier leg day, substituting deadlifts with:

Light deadlifts (5x8)
  *superset with*
Rope tucks (5x25)

Ideal conditions are for an ideal world. Still, sticking to the pre-scribed plan laid out by these orderly routines is very desirable. The body will respond to the consistent overload, the chemistry of the system (hormones, enzymes, metabolism, immune system) and desire become sharper and healthier; your psychological health and mental toughness improves big time. You're invested. You're cleaning out the attic and the junk from the trunk.

By now you should feel like a million bucks: stronger, energized, lighter, more toned, smiling and more certain.

## The Time-crunch Equalizer

A motivated, early trainee can perform a routine like the one that follows once he has dabbled with some consistency and intensity. Rely on your logic, and go at the pace and with the weights that are sufficient. Work up to three sets with a wise 7.5 intensity.

This is a pair of cute, cuddly workouts: cute as a rhino, cuddly as a shark. You should be well fueled before and after this bombardment. Are you drinking plenty of water?

### Day 1

Bench press (bar or dumbbell) (3-4x12, 10, 8, 6)
  *superset with*
Pulldowns (3-4x12, 10, 8, 6)

Dumbbell incline press (3-4-5x12,10, 8, 6)
  *superset with*
Pullovers (3-4x12,10, 8, 6)

Deadlifts (3-4x12, 10, 8, 6)

### Day 2

Barbell curls (3-4x12,10, 8, 6)
  *superset with*
Dips (3-4x10-12)

Leg extension (2-3x12)
  *tri-set with*
Leg curls (2-3x12, 10, 8)
  *and*
Calf raises (2-3x15-20)

Squats (3-4x15, 12, 12, 12)

I'm giving this routine an "A." Hit two, three or four total workouts a week, alternating continually. You might go heavy on muscle groups that lag and go light and quick on others for the happy pump. The pump may not build muscle, but it is rewarding and seductive. The regular demand on the vascular and cellular system contributes significantly to your ever-improving health. Aren't you the cool one?

# Leg Priority Training

Let's give legs priority once in a while. It's not unusual for men and women alike to undertrain their legs, assuming that running, biking or the StairMaster will be sufficient. Leg training ranks low on the popularity scale among weight-loss trainees. It's very hard work. Legs, the body's largest muscle group, put the greatest demands on the heart, lungs and vascular system. Not only exhausting, leg exercises are rather dull, limited in variation and cause a mean burn from major lactic acid accumulation. Basic torture. Early on it is enough to undertake the midsection, remain clothed in baggies or sweats while focused on the upper body mass. Don't look down. Can't see them. I'm busy.

Eventually, men and women do look down and strong legs are most desirable. They're exciting. Ask an older person and they'll tell you that if you lose your leg strength, you lose your mobility and independence. Legs are the foremost transporters, hikers, runners, dancers, and peddlers and are not that bad at kicking and jumping. They represent strength and impart power. They burn calories like crazy and make handy pants hangers.

I'm going out of my way to highly recommend squats to you who are overweight and under-muscled. You won't do them immediately, but plan on doing them someday soon when your conditioning is developed.

Squats are the foremost leg-and-glute muscle developers and large sums of calories are burned to build them and maintain them. Do I hear the fat burning? Your body will be stronger and more equipped to take on life with all its surprises. The abdominals, trunk, back and shoulders bear the strain and balance of the weighted bar and build muscle accordingly. Furthermore, with the body's largest muscles under overload, a message is sent to the brain that it must prepare itself for this increase of resistance by building proportionately the muscles of the whole system. The bones grow in density, balance is improved and the bottom and upper thighs are treated to the best lean-muscle workout money can't buy. Squats sizzle.

Are you ready? The leg routine you've been waiting for, leg priority, designed to fry fat and improve the form, function and power of the whole body:

Cardio warm-up
Crunches and leg raises

Leg extensions (4x12-15)
 *superset with*
Leg curls (4x8-12)

Squats—warm-up then 4x12 reps
(You can use other set and rep variations another time. We're
 here for life.)

Lunges (3x15)
 *fast-paced superset with*
Stiff-legged deadlifts (3x15)

Standing calf raise (4-5x15-25)
 *superset with*
Seated calf raise (4-5x15-25)

Volume plus volume equals volumes.

Begin with an aerobic warm-up followed by crunches and leg
raises. This is essential to energize the core muscles and joints, ready
the trunk, raise the heart rate, dispel distracting thoughts and focus
on the critical work ahead.

Start light to protect the joints and add weight each succeeding
set, working up to a moderate effort on the leg extensions. The powerful quad can too easily overload the knee, a joint already in a
compromised position. A slow tempo will accomplish more in the
extension with less risk, two seconds up, contract without hyper-ex-
tending for a sweet split-second and return over two seconds to the
start. No squealing. Once you're in condition, you can power into the
leg curl; a more explosive concentric with a slow eccentric. These
combined exercises increase circulation favorably and shape the quads,
hamstrings, glutes and calves while further preparing for the squats.

Squats deserve respect and require total concentration. Balance is critical with the knees and low back at risk. Practice strict form and proceed slowly with the weight you choose and you will be drawn to the whole-body work they provide. If possible, set up a rack and relax. For the first time squatter, safety bars can be placed at six or eight inches to allow short, yet effective, range of movement until strength and control are achieved. The bars can be lowered as confidence is raised.

Stand upright with the bar across your traps. Look forward and up a few degrees and squat down as if sitting on an imaginary chair, concentrating to push through your heels to ensure that the upper legs carry the workload. The more one descends, the more one tends to lean forward and force the resistance onto the lower back. Danger. Stay as upright as you can, continually holding the load on the quads. Do partial movements, and in time you'll achieve a full squat position with the thighs parallel to the floor, or deeper. Practice sessions should be performed with light weight, of course, yet too light a weight and you'll find it hard to maintain balance and locate a groove. Don't be shy.

Performed twice a week, this program has a long lifespan. The first day should be reserved for a heavy workout, with the second workout consisting of higher reps, less weight and increased pace to afford functional variety without overtraining.

## Virtue in abundance

Your training warehouse is well stocked; plans and blueprints are at your disposal with enough material and tools to build a castle. This is exciting. It's your castle, boss; let's get to work. Should you adorn yourself with wisdom and enthusiasm—most attractive and complimentary attire, indeed—you may throw caution to the wind. You're tough with a strain of spontaneity, proceeding one day at a time; determination without pressure, goals without deadlines, hopes without anxiety, first steps without fear, second steps without doubt, assessments without criticism, patience without frustration, discipline without captivity and healthy pride without conceit.

Have you ever made a list of virtues that you admire and wish existed in you? You've got them in abundance and are exercising them,

enlarging and polishing them and developing for them suitable companions here and now. Look around. You are a special person with
courage, fortitude and substance who knows why, where, when and
how to care for your health. You're remarkably different from the guy
and gal who plods along the common road. And as you continue
you'll distinguish yourself and simply appreciate the good work you've
chosen to do. I suspect you'll embrace exercise and sound eating like
the sunrise and the sunset.

# Chapter 22

## The Final Chapter:
### *In Closing*

Now what?

The information directly and indirectly related to the overweight condition, nutrition and exercise is vast. One door after another leads you through a maze of fascination and curiosity, questions, answers and puzzlement. Neat piles of printed copy from the Internet, stacks of purchased and borrowed books and a bulky file of printed email interviews surround me. I've learned a lot, and the research has been rewarding.

I have digested, compiled and summarized the material I thought would interest you and be of most value. It constitutes a small pond of knowledge upon the surface of which floats a comprehensive triangular distillation: exercise, eat right... always.

Very little of what was learned, I'm obliged to acknowledge, has had any bearing on my current exercising or eating regime nor has it pointed out a smarter way for me to go, were I to start all over again. The exploration only confirmed or clarified what my peers and I had been taught years ago or discovered along the path, a mixture of hand-me-down facts, logic, instinct and common sense... oh, yes, and consistent application—what you might call dedication or hard work.

My job has been to show you how to make fire and discover its elemental uses: cooking, warmth, light and safety. I have not shown you how to launch a blazing rocket ship. There's a list of references I recommend in the following pages that examine more deeply those burning details. Study the subject matter, write a thesis and acquire your degrees, but keep the practice simple and direct. It all comes down to honest exercise and food and an honest eye on your goal, one honest day after another.

Small changes in diet and exercise take you a long way in improving your health and performance and preventing the threat of obesity-related diseases. You who say no to junk food, walk by design with vim and vigor every day and lose 10 percent of your excess body weight are in the top quarter of the population who care for themselves. You have wisely removed yourself from harm's way. This is an attainable level of fitness. Bravo. But you won't stop there.

It seems to me that every conscious act we perform takes us closer to knowing who we are. I hope you know yourself better than you did before reading these pages. Where will you be next month? Where will you be a year from now? Your primary concern is self-preservation and that's a fact of life. I believe that to the degree that we care for ourselves, we love ourselves and are grateful for the precious gift of life. And it follows that to the degree we love ourselves, we can love others.

Those who neglect themselves, who take their life and health for granted, are a sad combination of arrogant, ignorant and slothful; they care little for themselves, hate too strong a word.

I'm not preaching world religion and peace through protein and weight lifting. I'm talking to you and encouraging a better, happier way of life by putting into effect one good training practice at a time at your own intelligent speed. Take each bad habit—one by one—and either remove it entirely or reduce it appropriately until it is no longer threatening.

Move forward always. Don't be weakened by what has been, looking back and regretting the past, judging yourself and carrying tiring emotional burdens. Press on toward the rewards that lie ahead. This act requires a maturity that grows at the very same time and from the same seed as the one you planted before picking up the book you have in your hands.

Don't be like so many who strike a match and let it burn down to their fingertips to go on in painful darkness. Light a candle, start a campfire, enjoy the warmth and see by the light. Shine.

• Read *Your Body Revival* entirely with an open mind, picking and choosing from the assortment of thoughts.

• Write down the date, a reference point to establish order—and consider keeping a training log.

• Intelligently see yourself as you would like to be.

• Recognize that changes—compromises—must be made.

• Be prepared to make the commitment to those changes, a strong statement of your character.

• Put the smaller-portion-yet-more-frequent eating plan into effect. This is a key factor and needs to be implemented over time. Relax and press on.

• Alter your balance of foods by lowering your sugar intake and increasing your protein intake. This is a second key factor. Take your time. Move forward.

• At the same time as you implement the dietary changes, begin a program of simple exercise: creative walking while planning further fitness activities. Exercise is the third key. Be strong and embrace its power.

• Pause amid your new practices to review them and generously reward yourself for the undertaking. You are not one of many who try; you are one of few who succeed. You are in the midst of your life and adding to it with an understanding and appreciation that has by many been buried under pleasure seeking and hidden by foolishness. Tell a friend; this is a mission.

• *Your Body Revival* is to serve you as a guide and future reference. Use it for motivation and assistance to hone your skills in training and eating. A dedication to health and strength will surface in you that will carry you forward at your own pace for a lifetime.

• The truth will be known to you only after devoted effort, the price tag placed on great and wonderful things. There is freedom in the restraints that bind you, the caring limitations you apply by your own wise and gentle hands. You are not taking on the habits of a monk or locking yourself in a cell. You are setting yourself free.

One day you will be able to broaden your margins—training limitations—if and when you choose, though few reformed participants care to let go of the good life. What appears to be rigid now will be preferable in the months to come and that which has devious appeal in your life today will likely lose its appeal by tomorrow. You'll miss payday sooner than miss a day at the gym. You'll eat tuna from the can rather than eat a hotdog on a bun. You'll crave the pump, burn and focus of a good workout over chocolate-cookie ice-cream cake.

Be heartened by the fact that there are no unturned stones. There are no secrets, no shortcuts or further facts hidden, obscure or forgotten that you need to know. The specific words required to define and convey the weight-loss process are somewhere among some 72,000 necessary to compile this book. I hope you had fun and learned something while uncovering them. More importantly, I hope you apply them with bountiful success.

God bless you.

*The end*
*&*
*the beginning*

# Glossary:
## *Weight Training Lingo*

**AEROBICS** *or* **AEROBIC EXERCISE**: any exercise that depends largely on the oxygen from the blood to fuel the energy production in the working muscles of the body. Examples are long-term endurance activities such as running, cycling and swimming.

**ANAEROBIC EXERCISE**: intense, short-burst exercise in which glucose and other cellular compounds energize the working muscle fibers exclusive of oxygen from the blood. Examples are weight lifting and sprinting.

**BARBELL** *or* **BB**: the main and basic implement of weight lifting (along with dumbbells) composed of a length of steel bar affixed with circular weights of differing denominations (plates) on both ends. Typical barbells are approximately one inch to one-and-an-eighth inches in diameter and five to seven feet long.

**BICEPS** *or* **BIs**: the muscles located on the front of the upper arm primarily engaged in bending the elbow. They pull and curl.

**BODYBUILDING**: the competitive sport or athletic hobby popularized over the last 60 years of the last century whose goal is to achieve muscular grandeur and symmetry through the activity of exercise (a.k.a. muscle building). The foremost activities to achieve bodybuilding perfection are weight lifting and resistance training through the application of a wide variety of gym equipment, cables and machines. Nutrition plays a major role in bodybuilding achievement.

**BURN**: the sensation of burning pain felt in the specific muscle or muscles under the intense contraction of resistance training. This reaction is due to the presence of lactic acid in the tissues, a byproduct of glucose metabolism during intense exercise. The burn, though painful, is welcomed by the trainee as the degree of burn endured indicates the level of muscle overload achieved, a key factor in muscle building. The burn is good, more is better.

**CARDIO**: pertaining to the heart. Exercise jargon for any effective aerobic activity.

**CONCENTRIC CONTRACTION**: the shortening of a muscle due to muscle contraction. Also known as the positive or positive contraction, moving the resistance away from the plane of gravity. For example, pulling the weight up in a biceps curl movement.

**DELTOIDS** *or* **DELTS**: the large, three-part muscles (front, side and rear deltoid) of the shoulder that move the arms away from the body. They push and press.

**DOMS**: recently popularized acronym for Delayed Onset Muscular Soreness, the phenomena of muscle soreness from sport or exercise afflicting the body a day or two after performance. Causes and desirability are subject to discussion.

**DUMBBELLS** *or* **DBs**: the short-handled partners of the barbell that complete the core of the weight lifting family. Dumbbells usually come in matching pairs and will range in length from six to eight inches (light DBs allowing for handgrip and a minimum of affixed plates) to 24 inches (heavy duty).

**ECCENTRIC CONTRACTION**: the lengthening of the muscle while under the tension of resistance. Also known as the negative or negative contraction, countering the resistance in its movement toward the gravity plane. For example, the lowering of the weight in a biceps curl.

**EXTENSION**: the straightening of a simple joint, as in the leg extension.

**EZ CURL BAR** *or* **BENT BAR**: a specially bent barbell to accommodate the handgrip, affording lifting and muscle-building advantages in both biceps curling and triceps extension exercises. Hand angles often protect wrists and elbows from abusive twist.

**FLOW**: a training term referring to the smooth, continuous movement from exercise to exercise without interruption in focus and action.

**FOCUS**: concentration on all the aspects of the work before you: muscles involved, the track they follow, the intensity of exertion, burn and pump, and signals of fatigue, injury or abuse. Concentration is extended to the weight used, technique applied, attitude, thirst, surrounding atmosphere, equipment and so on. Full-time job of primary importance.

**FULL RANGE OF MOTION**: a reference to the total action of a muscle(s) and the associated joint(s) in contrast to partial or abbreviated muscle and joint action.

**GETTING CUT**: bodybuilding term for gaining muscularity through serious application of training; exercise and diet without faltering.

**GETTING RIPPED**: bodybuilding slang for extreme muscularizing; gaining superior muscle hardness and definition through hard weight training and severe dieting.

**GLUTEUS MAXIMUS**: glutes, butt, bottom, rear. The outermost muscle of the three glutei found in each of the human buttocks.

**HAMSTRINGS** *or* **HAMS**: a.k.a the thigh biceps. Short for hamstring muscle, any of three muscles at the back of the thigh that function to flex and rotate the leg and extend the thigh.

**HIGH REPS**: terminology for a technique in muscle building where high repetitions (safe estimation: above 12) of given exercises are performed for specific purposes (exercise practice, muscle warm-up, injury repair, muscularity, sport conditioning, weight loss).

**HIT**: high-intensity training, a training technique where the trainee applies his training output to failure (extreme, maximum, total, dizzy, falling down—nausea is a good sign of the last rep) during each set after appropriately warming up. HIT workouts are typically shorter in duration and less frequent than other methods of training.

**INTENSITY**: extremity of strength, force, energy and feeling directed toward one's training. Combine with focus.

**ISOLATION**: a reference to exercising one specific muscle exclusive of others to focus effort on or protect that muscle.

**LACTIC ACID**: a byproduct of glucose and glycogen metabolism produced in the muscles during the hard work of exercise. Its presence is accompanied by muscle fatigue and burning pain. Embrace the pain and grow lean.

**LATISSIMUS DORSI** *or* **LATS**: the large muscles of the back that are chiefly responsible for the V-shape noticed in the male and female form. The lats are the prime movers for the adduction, extension and hyperextension of the shoulder joints. They pull; the shoulders push.

**LOW REPS**: the system of practicing low repetitions (below six) for specific effects in training (muscle mass, bulk, weight gain, power).

**MAX REP** *or* **SINGLES**: a reference in powerlifting to the heavy single repetition sets (single rep set) practiced in training to approach one's maximum (max) lifting output. 1RM= one rep max.

**MULTI-SET**: a series of exercises (usually 4 or 5) performed one after another with little pause. The total comprises one multi-set of perhaps 3, 4 or 5 multi-sets, the trainee in pursuit of specific goals (peak athletic conditioning, muscularity, aerobics, change of pace).

**OLYMPIC BAR and PLATES**: the popular weights used in competition and training. The standard bar weighs 45 pounds and is approximately seven feet long with rotating sleeves for lifting efficiency. Handsome tools.

**OLYMPIC LIFTING**: the weight-lifting sport of the Olympics, requiring enormous strength and extraordinary skill and athletics. It includes two lifts: the clean and jerk, and the snatch.

**PACE**: in weight lifting, as in other sports, a training term referring to the gauged speed at which one trains. Pace will vary with personality, purpose, mood or external factors (gym busy-ness, injury, other revolting interruptions).

**PECTORALS** *or* **PECS**: the broad band of muscles across the chest thats prime function is abducting the arms—moving the arms across the chest.

**PERSONAL TRAINER**: a private instructor to teach, assist and encourage a trainee of any sport at any level. Personal fitness instructors play an important role in the lives of many struggling and aspiring health- and condition-conscious people.

**POWERLIFTING**: the popular competitive sport of heavy weight lifting, which features the three power lifts: the bench press, the squat and the deadlift.

**PR**: abbreviation for personal record.

**PUMP**: muscle jargon referring to the enlarged and tightened sensation the lifter experiences within the working muscle resulting from the blood engorgement.

**PUMPING IRON**: originating in the '50s, slang for lifting weights.

**QUADRICEPS** *or* **QUADS**: the major four-part muscles of the front thighs primarily engaged in extending the leg at the knee.

**REPETITION** *or* **REP**: one complete movement of an exercise.

**RHYTHM**: a term an athlete uses to describe the sensation of flow and pace in his sport performance. The weight trainer's rhythm of training is achieved when functions are efficient and unimpeded.

**ROTATOR CUFF**: the complex of supporting and strengthening tendons and muscles that combine with the shoulder joint where the capsule of the shoulder and the head of the humerus (long bone of the upper arm) meet. A problem area for most active people, especially power athletes.

**SERRATUS**: the triple-tiered ridge of muscle located below the pecs and forward of the lats that accommodates the lats in adduction movement.

**SET**: the prescribed number of repetitions of any given exercise. Example: 1 set of 8 repetitions.

**SINGLE-SET TRAINING**: a system of training among strength lifters where sets of single repetitions are practiced with near-maximum output to develop skill, tenacity, structure strength and muscle power.

**SMITH PRESS**: a training apparatus that houses a bar that is smoothly guided by precision rods and bearings, allowing the trainee to press or squat with unique and purposeful advantage. Typically, plates are loaded as they are on free bars.

**SPECIALTY BARS and HANDLES**: some of the most effective pieces of equipment in the home or commercial gym are the assortment of various shaped bars and handles that effect and encourage hard training. They include the thick bar for grip development, the Buffalo bar for comfortable squat performance, the trap bar for back and leg building and the safety bar for dynamic and safe squatting. Handles for attachment to the cable devices come in a variety of lengths and bends and are made of steel, rope, leather or cloth. The right handles or bar for the right exercise or muscle development makes training fun and effective.

**SPLIT WORKOUT**: a workout divided into two or more parts thereby allowing different muscle groups to be worked at different times of the day (morning and evening) or on different days.

**SPOT**: the act of standing nearby in a supportive capacity as a co-lifter attempts heavy lifting where assistance might be required. The spot might include assistance in the case of failure to complete a lift, aid in bringing a heavy weight into starting position or added lifting help for an intense trainee forcing repetitions beyond his own limits.

**SPOTTER**: one who spots.

**SUPERSET**: two exercises performed alternately; one exercise followed by a second exercise in complement before resting, i.e. biceps curl followed by triceps extension equal one superset.

**TENDINITIS**: inflammation of a tendon, the tough band of connective tissue that connects a muscle to the bone. The affliction is common among athletes who strive hard or overtrain or allow themselves to get out of condition on occasion. Tendons, unfortunately, take a long time to heal. Ice often.

**TORSO**: the reference in *Your Body Revival* is to the trunk and midsection muscles: abdominals, obliques, erectors, intercostals.

**TRAINING LOG**: a book for recording training procedures and progress, exercises, sets, repetitions and weights used. Notations of observations, feelings and training responses often prove valuable at the moment of logging or in the future when comparisons and references guide the way.

**TRICEPS** *or* **TRIs**: the muscles on the back of the upper arm primarily for extending the elbow. They push or press.

**TRI-SETS**: three exercises executed one after the other in close succession, the total comprising one set, or tri-set.

**VOLUME**: a reference in muscle building to the total of sets and reps of exercises completed in a workout.

**VOLUME TRAINING**: the name of the technique where high volume is used.

**WORKOUT**: the noun; the sum total of one's time, collection of exercises performed and the energy burned on the gym floor, be it at the local gym or in your garage.

**WORKING IN**: the practice of cooperatively working with someone using a particular piece of equipment on the gym floor.

# RESOURCE APPENDIX

*in alphabetical order*

## BOOKS

## Nutrition & Diet Manipulation Books

Back to Protein: The Low Carb/
No Carb Meal Cookbook
Barbara Hartsock Doyen
ISBN: 0871319128

Bowes & Church's
Food Values of Portions Commonly Used
Jean Pennington, Anna De Planter Bowes,
Helen N Church
ISBN: 0397554354

Carbohydrate Addict's Lifespan Program,
The: A Personalized Plan for Becoming
Slim, Fit and Healthy in Your 40s, 50s, 60s
Dr. Rachael F. Heller, Dr. Richard F. Heller
ISBN: 0452278384

Carbohydrate Dieter's Diary, The
Corinne T. Netzer
ISBN: 0440508525

Complete Book of Food Counts, The
Corinne T. Netzer
ISBN: 0440225639

Everything You Need to Know
About Fat Loss
Chris Aceto
ISBN: 0966916824

Diet Cure, The: The 8-Step Program to
Rebalance Your Body Chemistry
Julia Ross
ISBN: 0670885932

First Place Member Kit:
The Bible's Way to Weight Loss
Carole Lewis
ISBN: 0830728694

Formula, The: A Personalized 40-30-30
Weight Loss Program
Gene Daoust, Joyce Daoust
ISBN: 0345443055

G-Index Diet. The: The Missing Link That
Makes Permanent Weight Loss Possible
Richard N. Podell William Proctor
ISBN: 0446365769

Glucose Revolution, The
Jennie Brand Miller
ISBN: 1569246602

Good Carb Cookbook, The: Secrets of
Eating Low on the Glycemic Index
Sandra Woodruff
ISBN: 1583330844

Insulin-Resistance Diet, The
Cheryle R. Hart M.D., Mary Kay Grossman
ISBN: 0809224275

Ironman's Ultimate Guide
to Bodybuilding Nutrition
Peter Sisco
ISBN: 0809228122

Ketogenic Cookbook, The
Dennis Brake, Cynthia Brake
ISBN: 1886559996

Ketogenic Diet, The: A Complete Guide
for the Dieter & Practitioner
Lyle McDonald
ISBN: 0967145600

Living Low-Carb: The Complete Guide to
Long-Term Low-Carb Dieting
Fran McCullough
ISBN: 0316557684

Low-Carb Cookbook, The: Complete
Guide to the Healthy Low-Carbohydrate
Lifestyle with over 250 Delicious Recipes
Fran McCullough, Michael & Mary Eades
ISBN: 0786862734

Manly Weight Loss: For Men Who Hate
Aerobics & Carrot-Stick Diets
Charles Poliquin, L. L. Dayton
ISBN: 0966275217

Menopause Diet, The
Larrian Gillespie
ISBN: 0967131707

Menopause Diet Mini Meal Cookbook
Larrian Gillespie
ISBN: 0967131715

Metabolic Diet, The
Mauro Di Pasquale
ISBN: 0967989604

Muscle Meals
John Romano
ISBN: 1889462012

Neanderthin: Eat Like a Caveman to
Achieve a Lean, Strong, Healthy Body
Ray V. Audette
ISBN: 0312243383

Nutrition Almanac (4th Ed)
Gayla J. Kirschmann, John D. Kirschmann
ISBN: 0070349223

Nutrition for Health, Fitness & Sport
Melvin H. Williams
ISBN: 0697295109

Outsmarting the Female Fat Cell : The First
Weight-Control Program Designed
Specifically for Women
Debra Waterhouse
ISBN: 0446675806

Outsmarting the Midlife Fat Cell : Winning
Weight Control Strategies for Woman over
35 to Stay Fit Through Menopause
Debra Waterhouse
ISBN: 0786884126

Protein Power: The High-Protein/Low
Carbohydrate Way to Lose Weight
Michael R. Eades, Mary Dan Eades
ISBN: 0553574752

Right Protein for Muscle & Strength, The
Michael Colgan
ISBN: 1896817092

Schwarzbein Principle, The: The Truth
About Weight Loss, Health and Aging
Diana Schwarzbein
ISBN: 1558746803

Sliced: State-Of-The-Art Nutrition for
Building Lean Body Mass
Bill Reynolds, Negrita Jayde
ISBN: 0809241161

Strong Women Eat Well : Nutritional
Strategies for a Healthy Body and Mind
Miriam E. Nelson
ISBN: 0399147403

Supercut:
Nutrition for the Ultimate Physique
Joyce L. Vedral, Bill Reynolds
ISBN: 0809253879

Ultimate Sports Nutrition
Frederick C. Hatfield
ISBN: 0809248875

Ultimate Sports Nutrition Handbook, The
Ellen Coleman, Suzanne Nelson Steen
ISBN: 0923521348

Week in the Zone, A
Barry Sears
ISBN: 006103083X

Women, Weight and Hormones
Elizabeth Lee Vliet, MD
ISBN: 0871319322

Zone, The: A Dietary Road Map to Lose
Weight Permanently
Barry Sears
ISBN: 0060391502

# Breakthrough Health Books

ACSM's Exercise Management for Persons
With Chronic Diseases & Disabilities
American College of Sports Medicine
J. Larry Durstine (Editor)
ISBN: 0873227980

Complete Book of
Vitamin and Mineral Counts, The
Corinne T. Netzer
ISBN: 0440223350

Complete Guide
to Vitamins, Minerals & Herbs
Art Ulene, M.D.
ISBN: 1583330046

Diabetes: Your Complete Exercise Guide
Neil F. Gordon
ISBN: 0873224272

Doctor's Guide to Weight Loss Surgery,
The: How to Make the Decision that Could
Save Your Life
Louis, Md Flancbaum, Erica Manfred
0971096805

Exercise, Nutrition & Weight Control
Perspectives in Exercise Science & Sports
Medicine, Vol 11
David R. Lamb (Editor)
ISBN: 1884125700

Exercise Physiology: Exercise,
Performance, and Clinical Applications
Robert A. Robergs, Scott O. Roberts
ISBN: 0815172419

Fats That Heal, Fats That Kill: Guide to Fats,
Oils, Cholesterol & Human Health
Udo Erasmus
ISBN: 0920470386

Heart Disease Breakthrough: The
10-Step Program That Can Save Your Life
Thomas Yannios, M.D.
ISBN: 0471353094

Metabolism at a Glance
J. G. Salway
ISBN: 0632052740

Nancy Clark's Sports Nutrition Guidebook
Nancy Clark
ISBN: 0873227301

Natural Hormonal Enhancement
Rob Faigin
ISBN: Not Available
www.extique.com

New Psycho-Cybernetics, The: The
Original Science of Self-Improvement
Maxwell Maltz, Dan S. Kennedy
ISBN: 0735202753

Realities of Nutrition
Ronald M. Deutsch, Judi Morrill
ISBN: 0923521259

Screaming to be Heard: Hormonal
Connections Women Suspect, and
Doctors Still Ignore
Elizabeth Lee Vliet, MD
ISBN: 0871319144

Strong Women—and Men—Beat Arthritis
Miriam E. Nelson
ISBN: 0399148523

Strong Women, Strong Bones: Everything
You Need to Know to Prevent, Treat, and
Beat Osteoporosis
Miriam E. Nelson
ISBN: 0399145974

Super T: The Complete Guide to Creating
an Effective, Safe & Natural Testosterone
Supplement Program
for Men and Women
Karlis C. Ullis, M.D.
ISBN: 0684863359

Syndrome X: Managing Insulin Resistance
Deborah S. Romaine, Jennifer B. Marks
ISBN: 0380814447

Syndrome X: The Complete Nutritional
Program to Prevent and Reverse Insulin
Resistance
Jack Challem, Burton Berkson, Melissa
Diane Smith
ISBN: 0471398586

Thyroid Power: Ten Steps to Total Health
Richard L. Shames, M.D., Karilee Halo
Shames, R.N., PH.D.
ISBN: 0688172369

Thyroid Solution, The
Ridha Arem, M.D.
ISBN: 0345429206

# Weight Training Books

Beyond Brawn: The Insider's ncyclopedia
on How to Build Muscle & Might
Stuart McRobert
ISBN: 9963616062

Body for Life:
12 Weeks to Mental & Physical Strength
Bill Phillips, Michael D'Orso
ISBN: 0060193395

Body Sculpting Bible for Men, The
Hugo Rivera, James Villepigue
ISBN: 157826085X

Body Sculpting Bible for Women, The
Hugo Rivera, James Villepigue
ISBN: 1578260868

Brother Iron, Sister Steel
A Bodybuilder's Book
Dave Draper
ISBN: 1931046654
www.davedraper.com

Challenge Yourself:
Leanness, Fitness & Health At Any Age
Clarence Bass
ISBN: 0960971475

Complete Book of Abs, The
Kurt Brungardt
ISBN: 0375751432

Complete Book of Butt and Legs, The
Kurt Brungardt, Mike & Brett Brungardt
ISBN: 0679754814

Cory Everson's Lifebalance: The
Complete Mind/Body Program
Cory Everson, Greta Blackburn
ISBN: 0399524444

Cory Everson's Fat-Free & Fit
Cory Everson, Carole Jacobs
ISBN: 0399518584

Fabulously Fit Forever
Frank Zane
ISBN: 1560251379

Getting Stronger:
Weight Training for Men and Women
Bill Pearl, D. Moran
ISBN: 0936070048

Insider's Tell-All Handbook
on Weight-Training Technique
Stuart McRobert
ISBN: 9963616097

Iron.Steel Training Log
Dave Draper
ISBN: 1931046530
www.davedraper.com

Ironman's
Ultimate Guide to Natural Bodybuilding
Peter Sisco (Editor)
ISBN: 0809228149

Lean for Life:
Stay Motivated & Lean Forever
Clarence Bass
ISBN: 0960971459

Lower Body Solution
Laura Dayton
ISBN: 0966275225

Muscle Mechanics
Everett Aaberg
ISBN: 0880117966

Optimum Power Program, The:
Your Personal Guide to Athletic Power
Michael Colgan
ISBN: 1896817009

New Encyclopedia of
Modern Bodybuilding, The
Arnold Schwarzenegger, Bill Dobbins
ISBN: 0684857219

Resistance Training Instruction
Everett Aaberg
ISBN: 0880118016

Sculpting Her Body Perfect
Brad Schoenfeld
ISBN: 0736001549

Serious Strength Training
Tudor O. Bompa, Lorenzo J. Cornacchia
ISBN: 0880118342

Strong Women Stay Slim
Miriam E. Nelson
ISBN: 0553379453

Strong Women Stay Young
Miriam E. Nelson
ISBN: 0553103474

Ultimate Fit or Fat: Get in Shape and Stay
in Shape With America's Best-Loved and
Most Effective Fitness Teacher
Covert Bailey
ISBN: 0618002049

## Flexibility Books

Beyond Stretching:
Russian Flexibility Breakthroughs
Pavel Tsatsouline
ISBN: 0938045180

Sport Stretch
Michael J. Alter
ISBN: 0880118237

Stretching (20th Anniversary Edition)
Bob Anderson, Jean Anderson
ISBN: 0936070226

Stretching Scientifically:
A Guide to Flexibility Training
Thomas Kurz
ISBN: 0940149303

Supple Body, The:
The Way to Fitness, Strength & Flexibility
Sara Black, Antonia Deutsch, Liliana
Djurovic
ISBN: 0028604415

# WEBSITES

## Diet, Health & Nutrition Sites

Alcoholism
www.alcoholism.about.com

Beverly International Nutrition
www.bodybuildingworld.com

Body For Life
www.bodyforlife.com

Calorie calculator, BMI calculator & more
www.practicalweightloss.com

Covert Bailey
www.covertbailey.com/articles.asp
Diabetes
www.diabetes.about.com

Diet & fitness logs and software online
www.dietpower.com
www.fitday.com
www.dakotafit.com
www.activelog.com
www.weightcommander.com

Dr. Pamela Peeke
www.drpeeke.com
www.fightfatafter40.com

Fad diet research
www.nutrition.about.com/msub4.htm

Fred Hatfield's ZigZag Diet
www.drsquat.com/articles/the_zigzag_diet.htm

General diabetes information
www.diabetes.org

Importance of water
www.members.aol.com/SaveMoDoe2/importance.htm
www.ag.arizona.edu/nsc/new/sn/hpwater.htm

Interactive menu planner
www.hin.nhlbi.nih.gov/menuplanner/menu.cgi

Low-carb diet FAQ
www.solid.net/~homerc

Medical information on obesity, weight
loss, eating disorders
www.weight.com

Menu and recipe analysis
www.dietsite.com

Nutrition
www.nutrition.about.com

Paleolithic Diet Page
www.paleodiet.com

Perimenopausal weight gain
www.nutrifit.org/nutr_info/midlife.html

Personalized diet and fitness counseling
www.ediets.com

Richard Simmons
www.richardsimmons.com

Stop smoking
www.quitsmoking.about.com

Sites on thyroid disease, chronic fatigue
and fibromyalgia
www.thyroid.about.com
www.chronicfatigue.about.com

TOPS Take Off Pounds Sensibly
www.tops.org

Tufts University nutrition website ratings
www.navigator.tufts.edu/index.html

Weight Commander Diet Software
www.interaccess.com/weightcmdr

Weigh Down Workshop
www.wdworkshop.com

Weight loss
www.weightloss.about.com

Weight loss facts and fiction
www.exrx.net/FatLoss/WeightLoss.html

Weight loss tips
www.100-weight-loss-tips.com

Weight loss tips and news
www.inch-aweigh.com

WeightWatchers Online
www.weightwatchers.com

## Weight Training Sites

Abdominal Training FAQ Page
www.timbomb.net/ab/ab.faq.html

Ageless Athletes
www.ageless-athletes.com

Clarence Bass' Ripped
www.cbass.com/index.htm

Dave Draper's IronOnline
www.davedraper.com

Dictionary of Lifting Terms and Techniques
www.trygve.com/weightsglossary.html

Exercise
www.exercise.about.com

Exercise Demonstrations & Calculators
www.biofitness.com/manual.html

Exercise glossary and instructions
www.exrx.net/Exercise.html

Internet Bodybuilding Search Engine
www.searchbodybuilding.com

Ironmind
Buffalo Bar, Apollon's Axle (Thick bar)
www.ironmind.com/main/index.asp

Manta Ray/Sting Ray Squat Assistance
www.adfit.com

Miriam Nelson's StrongWomen
www.strongwomen.com

Muscle & Fitness Online
www.muscleandfitness.com

PDA Piedmont Design Associates
Fractional Plates & Shrug bar
www.fractionalplates.com

Pendulum Fitness
www.pendulumfitness.com

Physique-Engineering Technologies
www.physique-engineering.com

PlateMate
www.theplatemate.com

PowerBlock dumbbell system
www.powerblocks.com

Shoulder Horn Rotator Cuff Repair
www.shoulderhorn.com

WeighTrainer
www.stas.net/weighttrainer/main.html

WeightsNet
www.weightsnet.com

Weight Training
www.bodybuilding.about.com

Weighty Matters Archive Page
staff.washington.edu/griffin/weights.html

Women's Weightlifting (Krista's Smash!)
www.stumptuous.com/weights.html

## Email Discussion & Support

Dave's IronOnline email discussion group
www.groups.yahoo.com/group/IronOnline

Dieter discussion group
www.dietersclub.com

Discussion of obesity surgery:

For those who have already had obesity
surgery
www.groups.yahoo.com/group/WLS-12StepRecovery
www.groups.yahoo.com/group/Bypass_Buddies
www.groups.yahoo.com/group/Graduate-OSSG

For those who are interested in obesity surgery
www.groups.yahoo.com/group/Fading-Away
www.dir.groups.yahoo.com/group/GastricBypass-InfoCentral
www.groups.yahoo.com/group/OSSG

Low-carb discussion groups
www.groups.yahoo.com/group/LOWCARB-BUDGET
www.groups.yahoo.com/group/CarbSmartRecipeExchange
www.groups.yahoo.com/group/low-carb-recipe-exchange
www.groups.yahoo.com/group/CelebrateLowCarb

## Research & Statistics

American Diabetes Association
www.diabetes.org

Ask the Dietitian
www.dietitian.com

Berkeley Heart Lab Advance Lipid Testing
www.berkeleyheartlab.com/services.html

Body Mass Index Table
www.nhlbi.nih.gov/guidelines/obesity/bmi_tbl.htm

Consumer Health Misinformation
www.quackwatch.com

Eating disorder information
www.nutrifit.org/nutr_info/nuted.html

Fast-food fact finder
www.olen.com/food

FDA Food safety, labeling, supplements
www.cfsan.fda.gov

Glycemic Index database
www.glycemicindex.com

Glycemic Index information page
www.mendosa.com/gi.htm

Kinesiology Forum
www.kines.uiuc.edu/kinesforum

Medline Medical & Scientific Research
www.medscape.com

Medline research
www4.infotrieve.com/newmedline/search.asp

National Center for Health Statistics
www.cdc.gov/nchs/fastats/overwt.htm

National Institute of Diabetes & Digestive & Kidney Diseases
www.niddk.nih.gov/index.htm

National Institutes of Health Osteoporosis Resource Center
www.osteo.org

National Library of Medicine Consumer Health Database
www.nlm.nih.gov/medlineplus

Nutrient Data Laboratory Food Composition Products
www.nal.usda.gov/fnic/foodcomp/Data/index.html

Nutrient information by name
www.nutrition.org/nutinfo

Obesity surgery,gastric by-pass, bariatric
www.asbs.org

Searchable calorie, protein, fat and carbohydrate charts
www.ntwrks.com/~mikev
www.rahul.net/cgi-bin/fatfree/usda/usda.cgi

Skeletal Muscles of the Human Body
www.ptcentral.com/muscles

Statistics and definitions related to obesity
www.niddk.nih.gov/health/nutrit/pubs/statobes.htm

USDA Food & nutrtion information center
www.nal.usda.gov/fnic/etext/fnic.html

USDA Nutrient Database
www.nal.usda.gov/fnic/foodcomp

## Email Newsletters & Print Journals

Dave's Weekly Email Newsletter
www,davedraper.com/
draper-newsletter.html

FDA Consumer
Superintendent of Documents
P.O. Box 371954
Pittsburgh, PA 15250-7954
$13.50, 6 issues
www.fda.gov/fdac/601_toc.html

Harcourt International Journal Publications
www.harcourt-international.com

Human Kinetics Publications
www.hkusa.com

Journal of Nutrition
American Society for Nutritional Sciences
9650 Rockville Pike
Bethesda, MD 20814

Larrian Gillespie's email newsletter
www.groups.yahoo.com/group/Larrian_Reports

Medical Journals Online
www.freemedicaljournals.com

Pounds Aweigh
PO Box 4731
Lancaster, PA 17604-4731
(877)840-1724
$15.95, 6 issues
www.poundsaweigh.com

Tufts University Health and Nutrition
Newsletter
P.O. Box 420235
Palm Coast, FL 32142-0235
(800)274-7581
$28.00, 12 issues
www.healthletter.tufts.edu

UC Berkeley Wellness Letter
Subscription Department
P.O. Box 420148
Palm Coast, FL 32142
(386)447-6328
$24.00, 12 issues
www.wellnessletter.com/index.html

University of Arizona
Online Nutrition, Exercise, and Wellness
Newsletter
//ag.arizona.edu/nsc/new/newsletter.htm

# *Index*

# Order Form

Your local bookstore can order *Your Body Revival* (ISBN: 1-931046-35-2) or *Brother Iron, Sister Steel* (ISBN: 1-931046-65-4) for you. If you are not near a bookstore, you may also order from the publisher direct, using our toll-free number, by fax, by mail or online at www.irononline.com.

Please send me the following:

\_\_\_\_ *Brother Iron, Sister Steel, A Bodybuilder's Book*, paperback
Personalized by Dave, $24.95 plus shipping ($3.95), total $28.90

\_\_\_\_ *Your Body Revival*, paperback
Personalized by Dave, $18.95 plus shipping ($3.95), total $22.90

California residents, please add 8% sales tax

TOTAL OF ABOVE    $_____

\_\_\_\_ BILL MY CREDIT CARD    or  \_\_\_\_ CHECK FOR $_____ IS ENCLOSED

Name on card: _____

Credit Card # &  expiration:_____

SPECIAL INSTRUCTIONS: To whom should Dave sign the book?

_____

NAME  _____

SHIPPING  ADDRESS_____

CITY, STATE, ZIP_____

_____

PHONE NUMBER (day)_____ (night)_____

Please fax or mail your order to the address or number below.
Thanks for your order!

On Target Publications
P O Box 1335, Aptos, Ca 95001
Toll-free (888) 466-9185 — Fax (831) 466-9183
**Visit us on the web at www.irononline.com**

# Order Form

Your local bookstore can order *Your Body Revival* (ISBN: 1-931046-35-2) or *Brother Iron, Sister Steel* (ISBN: 1-931046-65-4) for you. If you are not near a bookstore, you may also order from the publisher direct, using our toll-free number, by fax, by mail or online at www.irononline.com.

Please send me the following:

_____ *Brother Iron, Sister Steel, A Bodybuilder's Book*, paperback
    Personalized by Dave, $24.95 plus shipping ($3.95), total $28.90

_____ *Your Body Revival*, paperback
    Personalized by Dave, $18.95 plus shipping ($3.95), total $22.90

    California residents, please add 8% sales tax

TOTAL OF ABOVE    $_____

_____ BILL MY CREDIT CARD    or  _____ CHECK FOR $_____ IS ENCLOSED

Name on card: _____

Credit Card # & expiration:_____

SPECIAL INSTRUCTIONS: To whom should Dave sign the book?

_____

NAME  _____

SHIPPING  ADDRESS_____

CITY, STATE, ZIP_____

_____

PHONE NUMBER (day)_____ (night)_____

Please fax or mail your order to the address or number below.
Thanks for your order!

On Target Publications
P O Box 1335, Aptos, Ca 95001
Toll-free (888) 466-9185 — Fax (831) 466-9183
**Visit us on the web at www.irononline.com**

# Order Form

Your local bookstore can order *Your Body Revival* (ISBN: 1-931046-35-2) or *Brother Iron, Sister Steel* (ISBN: 1-931046-65-4) for you. If you are not near a bookstore, you may also order from the publisher direct, using our toll-free number, by fax, by mail or online at www.irononline.com.

Please send me the following:

\_\_\_\_ *Brother Iron, Sister Steel, A Bodybuilder's Book*, paperback
     Personalized by Dave, $24.95 plus shipping ($3.95), total $28.90

\_\_\_\_ *Your Body Revival*, paperback
     Personalized by Dave, $18.95 plus shipping ($3.95), total $22.90

     California residents, please add 8% sales tax

TOTAL OF ABOVE     $_____

\_\_\_\_ BILL MY CREDIT CARD     or \_\_\_\_ CHECK FOR $_____ IS ENCLOSED

Name on card: _____

Credit Card # & expiration:_____

SPECIAL INSTRUCTIONS: To whom should Dave sign the book?

_____

NAME   _____

SHIPPING  ADDRESS_____

CITY, STATE, ZIP_____

_____

PHONE NUMBER (day)_____ (night)_____

Please fax or mail your order to the address or number below.
Thanks for your order!

On Target Publications
P O Box 1335, Aptos, Ca 95001
Toll-free (888) 466-9185 — Fax (831) 466-9183
**Visit us on the web at www.irononline.com**

# Order Form

Your local bookstore can order *Your Body Revival* (ISBN: 1-931046-35-2) or *Brother Iron, Sister Steel* (ISBN: 1-931046-65-4) for you. If you are not near a bookstore, you may also order from the publisher direct, using our toll-free number, by fax, by mail or online at www.irononline.com.

Please send me the following:

_____ *Brother Iron, Sister Steel, A Bodybuilder's Book*, paperback
Personalized by Dave, $24.95 plus shipping ($3.95), total $28.90

_____ *Your Body Revival*, paperback
Personalized by Dave, $18.95 plus shipping ($3.95), total $22.90

California residents, please add 8% sales tax

TOTAL OF ABOVE    $_____

_____ BILL MY CREDIT CARD    or  _____ CHECK FOR $_____ IS ENCLOSED

Name on card:                   _____

Credit Card # & expiration:_____

SPECIAL INSTRUCTIONS: To whom should Dave sign the book?

_____

NAME  _____

SHIPPING  ADDRESS_____

CITY, STATE, ZIP_____

_____

PHONE NUMBER (day)_____ (night)_____

Please fax or mail your order to the address or number below.
Thanks for your order!

On Target Publications
P O Box 1335, Aptos, Ca 95001
Toll-free (888) 466-9185 — Fax (831) 466-9183
**Visit us on the web at www.irononline.com**